Man meets Microbes

An Introduction to Medical Microbiology

"To my Mother"

Acknowledgements

My thanks to my Mother, Mrs. Patricia Jamison for her encouragement; to Mrs. G. Dique, my typiste and Miss M. L. L. Gomes dos Santos, my artist, for their patient endurance; and to all those who taught me about Parasitology, Microbiology and Immunology.

Special thanks to Professor H. J. Koornhof for his constructive criticism of the manuscript.

Man meets Microbes

An Introduction to Medical Microbiology

by

Jennifer R. Jamison

MB, BCh, MSc, DTM & H, DPH

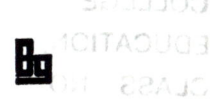

DURBAN
BUTTERWORTHS
1977

ISBN 0 409 085375

THE BUTTERWORTH GROUP

South Africa
BUTTERWORTH & CO (SA) (PTY) LTD
152-154 Gale Street, Durban 4001

England
BUTTERWORTH & CO (PUBLISHERS) LTD
88 Kingsway, London WC2B 6AB

Australia
BUTTERWORTHS PTY LTD
586 Pacific Highway, Chatswood, Sydney, NSW 2067

Canada
BUTTERWORTH & CO (CANADA) LTD
2265 Midland Avenue, Scarborough, Ontario M1P 4S1

New Zealand
BUTTERWORTHS OF NEW ZEALAND LTD
26-28 Waring Taylor Street, Wellington

USA
BUTTERWORTHS (PUBLISHERS) INC
19 Cummings Park, Woburn, Massachusetts 01801

Printed in South Africa by
INTERPRINT (PTY) LTD, DURBAN

Preface

Man lives in a world teeming with life. Much of this activity is invisible to the naked eye. 'Man meets Microbes' is the story of the interaction between man and this 'invisible' world. The tale is one of co-operation and conflict, of détente and the cold war. 'Man meets Microbes' is an account of success and failure as man and microbes strive towards peaceful co-existence.

June, 1977   JENNIFER JAMISON
Johannesburg

v

Foreword

With the advent of new diploma and degree courses in the rapidly developing fields of Nursing, Nursing Education and the allied medical disciplines, the need for a microbiology textbook which caters specifically for paramedical students is obvious. Dr. Jennifer Jamison's keen interest in health education and her experience as a lecturer in clinical microbiology to medical students, technologists and nurses makes her an eminently suitable person for the task of writing such a textbook.

In "Man meets Microbes" the close association between man and his micro-organisms is stressed. As much attention is given to the host's responses to infecting organisms as to the agents themselves. The importance of performing the correct procedures to make a microbiological diagnosis is emphasized. The book contains a wealth of essential information on medical microbiology presented in a refreshingly direct and easily assimilable form. It could be read and studied to advantage not only by nurses but also by technologists, interns and other students of medical and allied disciplines.

It is my hope that students will enjoy the author's easy conversational style and the simple yet striking presentation of summaries, tables and illustrations as much as I did.

PROFESSOR H. J. KOORNHOF
MB ChB (Cape Town) DCP Dip Bact FRC Path (Lond)

Sterilisation
195

Immunity
12 – innate ✓
19 ×
37 ✓
38 (✓)
171 ×
192

Contents

Contents

List of Tables

List of Figures

Recommended Reading

BOCOCK, E. J.   *Microbiology for Nurses*, Balliére, Tindall and Cassell Ltd., London, 1969, 3rd ed.

CRUICKSHANK, R. *et al. Medical Microbiology*, vol. 1, Churchill Livingstone, London, 1975, 12th ed.

GILLIES, R. R. and Dodds, T. C.   *Bacteriology Illustrated*, Churchill Livingstone, London, 1973, 3rd ed.

JAWETZ, E. *et al.   Review of Medical Microbiology*.   Lange Medical Publications, Los Altos, Calif., 1976, 12th ed.

NETER, E.   *Medical Microbiology*, F. A. Davis, Philadelphia, 1966, 5th ed.

CHAPTER 1

General Introduction

A knowledge of organisms capable of causing disease in man is an essential part of any course concerned with the health of man. Infective organisms take their place high on mortality and morbidity lists. Factors causing disease in man are divided into two large groups — Congenital and Acquired. The acquired group of diseases is by far the larger group. Congenital defects can and do affect the course of acquired diseases. A congenital defect in the host's immune system may permit easier entrance and proliferation of an infective agent.

Acquired disease is commonly classified under the following headings:
> Traumatic
> Infective
> Neoplastic
> Degenerative
> Metabolic

In any single individual, factors attributable to one or more of these causes may be operating at any one time.

This book is concerned with the infective aspects of disease in man. It considers the role of organisms in causing disease. It is also concerned with the response to, and defence of man against these organisms. Hospital acquired infections and the role played by the nursing staff in either spreading or controlling these outbreaks are also discussed. The prevention and control of disease is considered from both the general and nurses' point of view.

Nurses have an important rôle to play in the prevention and control of nosocomial infections. A knowledge of micro-organisms, their mode of spread, their interaction with different hosts and their susceptibility to physical and chemical agents is an essential part of the nurse's armamentarium in combating infectious disease.

THE HISTORY OF MICROBIOLOGY

Centuries ago man believed in spontaneous generation. He ascribed epidemics to poisonous vapours created by disturbances within the earth and on other planets. Today man believes in microbiology. He believes in fungi, in bacteria, in viruses and in immunology. He knows how to treat and also how to prevent many infectious diseases. This change from fantasy to fact is attributable to the work of many men. Some of the "greats" will be mentioned.

Antony van Leeuwenhoek (1632-1723), a cloth merchant in Delft, Holland, designed a microscope with specially ground lenses. His microscope could magnify up to 300 times. The ability to see what was previously "invisible", to visualize organisms never seen by the naked eye, was a major advance. Microscopy remains a cornerstone in the identification of micro-organisms. Today man, with improved lenses and energy or light sources, uses microscopy routinely in the everyday handling of specimens from patients.

In vitro growth and multiplication of Van Leeuwenhoek's "animalicules" was a vital step in the advance of microbiology. Spallanzani, an Italian priest (1729-1799), introduced the use of sterile culture media. He also showed that boiling could kill organisms and hence render articles 'sterile'. The ability of heat to destroy micro-organisms was confirmed by Schwann in 1837. John Tyndall (1877) found that certain micro-organisms could resist boiling. This resistant form was described by Ferdinand Cohen as an endospore — a stage in the life cycle of *Bacillus subtilis*. Tyndallization or intermittant sterilization is a method of destroying spores.

Interest in three different aspects of microbiology has developed into three disciplines. Industrial microbiology has evolved out of the initial observation that certain organisms can ferment carbohydrates. Agricultural microbiology is related to the cycle of organic matter in nature, and medical microbiology is the study of disease in man caused by microorganism. The new science of medical microbiology was founded mainly due to the contributions made by Pasteur and Koch.

Fracastorius of Verona in 1546 suggested that disease could be spread from one person to another either directly or via fomites. Robert Koch (1876) was a country doctor in Germany. He was able to show that a square bacillus was present in the blood of all the animals dying of anthrax. His experience with anthrax and tuberculosis led him to outline the famous Koch's postulates in 1884. Koch's postulates must be fulfilled before a specific micro-organism can be accepted as the cause of a specific disease. Koch's postulates require

(*a*)   that the organism be present in the tissue of the infected animal;

(*b*)   that this organism be grown in artificial culture;

(*c*)   that the organism from (*b*) on introduction into a susceptible host is capable of inducing that specific disease in this host; and,

(*d*)   that the organism should be present in and be cultured from the lesion induced in the susceptible animal host (*c*).

During the last quarter of the 19th century many of the organisms causing serious disease in man were identified. Between 1879 and 1889 the German School isolated the organisms causing diphtheria, typhoid, cholera, tuberculosis, tetanus, gonorrhoea and meningococcaemia. The pneumococcus, staphylococcus and streptococcus were also isolated. These advances were made possible due to the many technical advances in the staining and microscopy of micro-organisms. The use of solidified culture media also facilitated the growth of pure cultures. Koch was the key figure in these advances.

It was the 19th century that saw the introduction of antiseptic technique. Joseph Lister (1867), the English surgeon, was convinced that living organisms were responsible for the gangrene and septicaemia suffered by his patients. Wounds were kept sterile using carbolic acid treatment topically and phenol dressings. Semmelweis (1848) in Vienna showed that hand washing in chloride of lime could decrease the puerperal sepsis rate. Prior to this students, interns and obstetricians had moved freely between the post-mortem room and the labour ward. Semmelweis's handwashing procedure reduced the rate of puerperal sepsis. In Semmelweis's hands case fatalities due to puerperal sepsis in those women reaching hospital decreased from 8,3% to 2,3%.

Transmission of disease plays an important role in medical microbiology. Today airborne spread of organisms may still be excluded from containers by cottonwool plugs. These plugs were introduced in the first half of the 19th century by Schroeder and Van Dusch. John Hunter (surgeon) inoculated himself with the purulent exudate from a patient suffering from gonorrhoea thereby transmitting this disease (plus syphilis) from the patient to himself. John Snow in 1854 traced a localized cholera epidemic to a street pump. He surmised that cholera was a disease spread by faecally contaminated water.

Prevention of disease is not only practised by preventing the introduction of organisms into the host, it can also be practised by stimulating the host's immune response. Stimulation of the host's response is achieved by vaccination. Vaccination was introduced by Edward Jenner in 1796. He took material from the rash on the arm of a dairy-maid suffering from cowpox. This infectious material he then inoculated into an 8 year old boy; on subsequent exposure to small-pox the boy remained healthy! The rhyme referring to the pretty milk maid may not have been meant as a compliment to her features but rather to her skin. The clear complexion of milk-maids was thanks to their resistance against the scars caused by smallpox — the occupational hazard of cowpox made them immune to the smallpox virus. Pasteur in 1881 inoculated sheep against anthrax. He discovered 4 methods of attenuating organisms. His methods consisted of —

- (*a*) ageing the culture
- (*b*) drying the culture
- (*c*) passaging the organism through another less susceptible host species
- (*d*) growing the organism at high temperatures.

The era of active treatment using drug therapy began with Ehrlich's "magic bullet". He and Hata introduced an organic arsenical (606) for the treatment of syphilis. This was named 606 as the previous 605 substances tried had failed. Drug therapy for infectious diseases took another major step forward with Flemming's pioneering work in discovering penicillin.

Domagh in 1930 introduced prontosil — the fore-runner of sulphona-mides. Nobel prizes have been awarded to Domagh and also to Flemming, Florey and Chain. The latter two workers purified and concentrated peni-cillin making it a drug which could be available to all mankind.

Viruses are smaller than bacteria — in fact the original definition of a virus was an infectious agent capable of passing through a bacterial filter. Later their absolute requirement for an intra-cellular environment was recognised and this criterion was added to the original definition. Plant viruses were discovered in 1892, and in 1900 a virus causing human disease was found, viz. the yellow fever virus. It was in 1949 that Enders, Weller and Robbins showed that the polio virus could be grown on cell or tissue culture. The identification, growth and description of viruses is thus an achievement of the 20th century.

LOUIS PASTEUR — 'THE FATHER OF MODERN BACTERIOLOGY'

Pasteur, a French chemist, became interested in bacteriology due to a request to investigate the cause of faulty fermentation of wine (1856). His inquiries into the process of fermentation led him to suggest that fermen-tation was a living process. He found that different substrates encouraged the growth of different organisms and led to different end product pro-duction, e.g. either lactic acid or alcohol may be formed. Today selective culture media are widely used in bacteriology laboratories. Pasteur was also the first person to suggest that life could exist in the absence of air. Prior to Pasteur anaerobic organisms were not suspected.

Pasteur contributed to the following aspects of microbiology —

(a) He dealt a blow to the concept of spontaneous generation.

(b) He established a new field — that of microbial metabolism.

(c) He was the first to accept anaerobic growth.

(d) He established the role of micro-organisms in the transmission of disease.

(e) Pasteurization is today a password in milk processing. The idea originated from the introduction, by Pasteur, of gentle heating into the beer and wine industry.

(f) Pasteur extended Jenner's work and introduced the concept of immunization with live attenuated organisms.

(g) The concept of utilizing selective living tissue for the cultivation of organisms was introduced by Pasteur during his work with the virus causing rabies. He took an extract from the brain of a fatal case of rabies and injected this into the brain of a dog. The dog became rabid. Pasteur failed to recognise that rabies was caused by a non-bacterial agent.

PRELIMINARY CLASSIFICATION

Parasites and micro-organisms capable of causing disease in man are found classified amongst the Kingdoms Animalia and Protista. Viruses, the smallest of the agents capable of infecting man, are classified in a different group.

KINGDOM: *ANIMALIA*

Certain of the worms in this kingdom are capable of causing disease in man. Two groups or phyla are of significance to man's health.

(*a*) *The Platyhelminths* (flat worms)

This phylum includes:
  (1) The Trematodes (Flukes):
    The blood fluke — Schistosome/Bilharzial fluke
    The liver flukes — Fasciola and/or Clonorchis (The Chinese liver fluke)
    The lung fluke — Paragonimus
  (2) The Cestodes (tape worms)
    Included in this group are the following tape worms —
    The beef tape — *Taenia saginata*
    The pork tape — *Taenia solium*
    The fish tape — *Diphyllobothrium latum*
    The dog tape — *Diphyllidium caninum*
    Hydatid disease is included in this group: the worm involved is *Echinococcus granulosus*.

(*b*) *The Nematodes* (round worms)
    Hookworms — Ancylostoma and Necator
    The ascarids of man — *Ascaris lumbricoides*
    The ascarids of dogs — *Toxocara canis*
    The ascarids of cats — *Toxocara catti*
    The whipworm — *Trichuris*
    The pinworm — *Enterobius*

A superfamily in this phylum are the filarial worms. This group of nematodes is important in the tropics. Different members of the filaria cause 'river blindness', 'elephantiasis' and 'calabar swellings'.

The Arthropoda

Within the kingdom *Animalia* a large group of creatures fall in the phylum arthropoda. The arthropods are those animals which have jointed appendages and a chitinous exoskeleton. Their role in infectious diseases of man is that of a vector or intermediate host. Arthropods may act as hosts to certain micro-organisms — in fact certain micro-organisms may require a period of development in an arthropod in order to complete their life-cycle, e.g. the organism causing malaria in man requires a period of development in the mosquito. These infected arthropods are then capable of transmitting the micro-organisms to man. Other arthropods may act as mechanical vectors of disease — these arthropods are not infected by the micro-organism, they merely transport the organism, e.g. the house fly may settle on faeces and pick up shigella bacilli or the poliovirus on its feet. Certain arthropods are themselves capable of causing infestations in man.

They may act as ecto-parasites, e.g. scabies is caused by *Sarcoptes scabiei*, an arthropod.

The kingdom of *Animalia* is composed of a large number of different members. All these members are multicellular creatures. The basic unit — the cell — is specialized in these animals to form groups of specialized cells. Groups of specialized cells form organs systems — each organ system is modified to fulfil a specific function. The kingdom of *Animalia* is composed of complex, and has relatively highly evolved members, e.g. man himself.

KINGDOM: *PROTISTA*

The kingdom of *Protista* is divided into two large groups — the higher protists and the lower protists.

Higher protists

These protists have eukaryotic cells. This cell type is similar to that found in man and animals. Protozoa and fungi are the two groups of higher protists capable of causing disease in man.

The Protozoa

These are unicellular (acellular) organisms. Protozoa house all the machinery necessary for life and reproduction in a single cell. The protozoa may be divided according to their means of locomotion — the amoebae move by producing cytoplasmic protrusions — pseudopodia, *Balantidium coli* moves using cilia while the flagellates use their flagellae. The flagellates may be further divided into blood and tissue flagellates. The blood flagellates, e.g. trypanosomes are found in the blood of their host. In order for trypanosomes to infect a new host they require the assistance of an arthropod vector. Leishmanial organisms are also flagellates requiring an arthropod vector. *Trichomonas* and *Giardia* are tissue flagellates found in the genital or gastro-intestinal tract. These tissue flagellates can spread from host to host without the assistance of any arthropod vector. Certain protozoa lack locomotory organelles, e.g. *Toxoplasma* and *Plasmodium* (the organism responsible for malaria).

The Fungi

Previously classified in the plant kingdom the fungi are now classed as higher protists. They lack chlorophyll and are not differentiated into leaves, stems or roots. Two varieties of fungi are found — a filamentous branching form and a round or ovoid unicellular form. The filamentous form consists of hyphae which are collectively called a mycelium. The unicellular form are yeast-like organisms. In certain groups of fungi both of these forms may be found — these groups are referred to as dimorphic fungi.

Fungi are assuming increasing importance in medicine since man has entered the age of organ transplantation and cancer therapy. Fungi take advantage and cause disease in man when his defence against disease is lowered. Fungi are particularly pathogenic to man when medical science is manipulating his immune system.

Lower protists

The prokaryotic cell type is found in this group. These cells differ from those of man in certain important respects — a knowledge of these differences plays an important rôle in the basis of treatment of diseases caused by these organisms. Many of the common important pathogens are found amongst the lower protists —

> Bacteria
> Mycoplasma
> Chlamydia
> Rickettsia

The last two groups mentioned are obligate intracellular parasites, they are incapable of multiplication and growth outside of a host cell.

KINGDOM: THE VIRUSES

Viruses are classified according to the type of nucleic acid they contain. If the virus contains deoxyribo-nucleic acid it is classified as a DNA virus; if it contains only ribonucleic acid, as a RNA virus. Further classification depends on the nucleic acid present having a single or double strand. Certain viruses, in addition to containing a nucleic acid strand surrounded by a polypeptide coat, the capsid, have an outer lipid membrane. Viruses with a lipid membrane are said to be enveloped. Enveloped viruses are sensitive to ether.

The infectious particle is termed a virion. When a virion infects a host cell it sheds its protective capsid. Multiplication of the virus inside the host cell consists of replication of its nucleic acid. The genetic information about how to produce more viruses is contained on the nucleic acid. The virus enters the host cell, adapts to the new environment and takes control of that cell's enzymatic and synthetic machinery. Viral nucleic acid converts host cells into virus producing factories.

Table I
A PRELIMINARY CLASSIFICATION

KINGDOM	MEDICAL IMPORTANCE	TYPICALLY
Animalia	worms vectors of disease intermediate hosts	Multicellular
Protista		Unicellular
Higher Protists	Protozoa, e.g. organisms causing malaria, amoebiasis Fungi, e.g. organisms causing ringworm	
Lower Protists	Bacteria Rickettsia Chlamydia Mycoplasma	

Viruses	Small intracellular parasites not
	  classified in any of the recognised
	  kingdoms.
		Sub-cellular

Table II

DIFFERENCES BETWEEN BASIC CELL TYPES

The Eukaryotic Cell	The Prokaryotic Cell
(a more advanced cell type)	(a more primitive cell type)

A. NUCLEIC ACID

Genetic information

Nucleus — consisting of:	Nucleoid — consisting of:
DNA arranged as chromosomes within a nuclear membrane.	A single coiled molecule of double stranded DNA attached at one point to the cytoplasmic membrane. No nuclear membrane is present.

Staining

Basic proteins present — histones are basic polyamines which are stained by standard dyes used in histology.	DNA is not bound to basic proteins thus special staining techniques are required.

Replication

Mitosis and meiosis	Binary fission and growth

B. CYTOPLASM

1. Metabolism

(a) Enzymes for oxidative phosphorylation — the cytochromes associated with electron transfer and the respiratory chain.

Found in mitochondria — cell membrane bound organelles.	Found as part of cytoplasmic membrane.

(b) Protein synthesis — The ribosome sedimentation constant:

80s	70s
(components $= 40s + 60s$)	(components $= 30s + 50s$)

   i.e. there is a difference in ribosomal structure between cells of different types.

(c) Metabolic pathways for vitamin synthesis, e.g. enzymes required for the synthesis of folic acid from para-amino benzoic acid

absent	present

2. Physical and Chemical Characteristics

Extensive membrane bound system in the cytoplasm	absent
Cytoplasmic motility — amoeboid movement cytoplasmic streaming vacuole activity (formation, migration, streaming).	absent

C. THE OUTER LAYER — i.e. the layer between cytoplasm and the external environment.

(a) The cytoplasmic membrane —

Lipoprotein and cholesterol	Lipoprotein
	Multiple enzyme systems associated with the cytoplasmic membrane.

(b) The cell wall —

Lacking in animal cells. Higher protists may have a polysaccharide cell wall of, e.g. chitin or cellulose	Multilayered cell wall lipopolysaccharide lipoprotein murein/peptidoglycan techoic acid.
	A capsule may also be present.

DIFFERENCES BETWEEN BASIC CELL TYPES

The Eukaryotic Cell	The Prokaryotic Cell

D. SPECIALISED STRUCTURES

(a) Organelles of locomotion — these cells may be non-motile or display motility due to —	
Cilia	
Flagella	Flagella
Cytoplasmic streaming — pseudopodia	
(b) Other —	Pili may function in various ways, e.g. adhesion conjugation

E. EXAMPLES

Animal cells, Protozoa, Fungi.	Bacteria, Rickettsiae.

The value of being familiar with the differences between the different cell types

(1) Recognition of different physical characteristics aids in the separation of organisms not only into basic cell types but also into more specific groupings.

(2) In the treatment of disease caused by an infecting organism drug therapy must be directed at inherent differences between the organism and the host. The concept of differential toxicity is based on physical and/or chemical properties possessed by only one member in a host-parasite relationship. To kill the organism without causing damage to, or death of, the host, it is necesaary to interfere with the cellular machinery of the organism and not with that of the host.

CHAPTER 2

Host-parasite Relationships

INFLAMMATION AND INFECTION

Inflammation is the local response of living tissue to injury. This injury must be sub-lethal. If the injury is too severe, cell death — necrosis — results. Inflammation is characterised by redness, heat, swelling, pain and loss of function. Chemical mediators include serotonin, histamine, brady-kinin, the breakdown products of complement, and nucleic acids. Cells involved in inflammation include:

Polymorphonuclear leucocytes

(a) Neutrophils — these highly mobile cells have a short life of only a few days. They are specialized in phagocytosis. The release of their lysosomal enzymes into areas of inflammation leads to tissue diges-tion and pus formation.

(b) Eosinophils — these are associated with allergic types of inflam-mation and parasitic infections.

(c) Basophils — these cells play an important role in the initiation of inflammatory changes. They release chemical mediators of inflam-mation, e.g. histamine, serotonin, and heparin.

Monocytes — in blood ⎫ These phagocytes are less active than neu-
Macrophages — in tissue ⎬ trophils but have a longer life span of weeks
⎭ or months.

Lymphocytes — These are immunologically competent cells with a select role in host defence.

The body responds to any form of injury with inflammation. When the insult is associated with an organism this 'injury' is termed infection. Depending on the type of organism involved the infection may be acute, in which case polymorphs are the predominant cells; or it may be chronic in which case mononuclear cells (macrophages) predominate. In infection both the host's defences and the method whereby the organism causes disease, are important. Infection is thus inflammation plus an organism. Inflammatory responses depend only on the host; response to infection is determined by interaction between the host and the infecting organism. Host-parasite interaction determines the outcome of an infectious disease.

HOST-PARASITE RELATIONSHIPS

There is a constant interaction between man and his environment. Man lives in an environment in which micro-organisms abound. Certain of these organisms are harmless saprophytes, others cause disease. Those that cause disease fall into two groups —

(*a*) those that always cause disease — pathogens;

(*b*) those that only sometimes cause disease — potential pathogens.

If indigenous micro-organisms, sometimes called commensals, are introduced into a normally sterile site of the host's body, or if the host's defences are depressed, then the organism can cause disease. Potential pathogens taking advantage of a change in this host's immunity are termed opportunists. The infection so caused is an opportunistic infection.

Table III
EXAMPLES OF POTENTIALLY PATHOGENIC ORGANISMS CONSTITUTING PART OF THE NORMAL FLORA

The gastro-intestinal tract	Transfer to other sites may result in:
Clostridium perfringens	Gas gangrene
Streptococcus faecalis	Urinary tract infection, endocarditis
Escherichia coli	Urinary tract infection
Anaerobes — Bacteroides	
Fusobacterium	Wound sepsis, Puerperal sepsis, etc.
Peptococci	
Peptostreptococci	
Candida	Candidosis
The vagina	
Clostridia	Gas gangrene
Listeria	Neonatal meningitis
Group B streptococci (*Strep. agalactiae*)	Neonatal meningitis and septicaemia
Anaerobic streptococci	Abscess formation

The study of host-parasite relationships is the study of the interaction between man and a variety of organisms. This interaction is constant and

Figure 1
THE HOST-PARASITE SEESAW

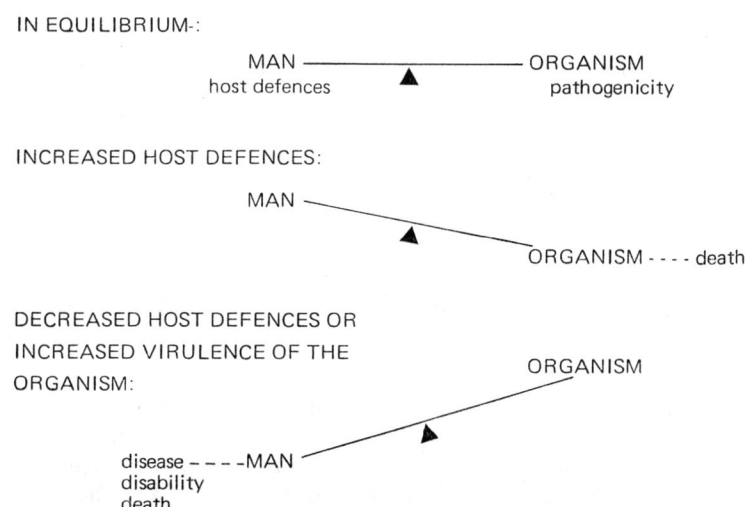

IN EQUILIBRIUM-:

MAN ——————— ORGANISM
host defences   pathogenicity

INCREASED HOST DEFENCES:

MAN
ORGANISM - - - - death

DECREASED HOST DEFENCES OR INCREASED VIRULENCE OF THE ORGANISM:

ORGANISM

disease - - - -MAN
disability
death

variable. Man's defence mechanisms are poised against the ability of the organism to multiply and cause disease. An upset in the equilibrium between man and the organism results in either disease, disability or death of man; or in the death of the organism.

THE HOST

The host's defence against disease depends upon:

A. Non-specific defences   (a) Superficial barrier
                                         (b) Second line defence

B. Specific defences   (a) Humoral immunity
                                         (b) Cellular immunity

Local factors, e.g. a poor blood supply to an area, or general factors, e.g. poor nutrition, will modify the non-specific and also the specific host defences.

A.   NON-SPECIFIC DEFENCES

These general defences are also termed innate immunity. They are present in all healthy people and their efficiency may be altered by various host factors. Age, nutrition, sex, the gene composition, and endocrine balance all influence the individual's non-specific defence against infection. The very old and the very young are more prone to infection than adolescents or adults. Most subclinical infections occur in the 2-15 year age group.

The diabetic is more at risk of infection than the non-diabetic. The patient with peripheral vascular disease is at greater tisk of being unable to cope with an infection of an ischaemic limb or digit than the individual with a normal blood supply. The malnourished patient is at risk of infection as his superficial defences and his immune responses are impaired. In the malnourished patient gastro-enteritis may be fatal.

The organism in order to infect the host must penetrate the superficial barrier. Once the superficial barrier has been impaired the organism can attempt to establish itself by multiplication. A compromised superficial barrier leads to interaction between the host and the organism.

(a) SUPERFICIAL BARRIER

The superficial barrier consists of three parts:

(1) The mechanical barrier

This provides a barrier to organisms only for as long as the barrier is physically and functionally intact. Examples of the mechanical barrier include:

    (i) An intact skin and mucous membrane lining. Skin is composed of keratinized epithelium. It subjects organisms to drier conditions than does mucous membranes. Many Gram-negative bacilli can be killed by drying. Organisms are shed from the skin surface as desquamation takes place. Certain organisms only infect superficial keratinized tissues, e.g. the dermatophytes (ringworm). Occasionally bacteria are capable of attaching to the epithelial cells of mucous membranes, e.g. gonococci attach to the urethral cells via pili; entero-pathogenic *E.coli* differ from non-pathogenic *E.coli* in their increased ability to attach to the mucosal surface of an infant's intestine.

(ii) The respiratory escalator. The respiratory tract is lined by a thin film of mucus. The cilial action of specialized cells found in the respiratory tract moves this mucus layer from the deeper portions of the respiratory tree to the pharynx. Bacteria and other particles trapped by the sticky mucus are moved out of the respiratory tract. This mechanical escalator is formed by the action of the cilia in the mucus layer.

(iii) A urinary lavage. The distal portion of the urethra is colonized by bacteria. The bladder is sterile. Urine, a sterile fluid, is expelled from the bladder to the exterior via the urethra. The urine passing down the urethra flushes bacteria out of the urethra.

(2) The chemical barrier

Secretions from various parts of the body contain a variety of chemical substances capable of interfering with the growth and multiplication of a variety of organisms.

(i) Certain of the fatty acids secreted in sebum by the sebaceous glands are toxic to fungi. It is postulated that the endocrine or hormone balance affects the secretion of these saturated toxic fatty acids — this may account for the resistance against ringworm which is acquired after puberty.

(ii) Tears, a lubricant solution containing chemical substances active against bacteria, rinse the eye with each blink. Lysozyme, an important constituent of tears, acts on the cell wall of Gram-positive bacteria rendering the bacterium susceptible to lysis.

(iii) The stomach barrier. Food, acceptible by public health standards, may contain up to 10^7 organisms per gram. This food with its bacterial population is ingested and reaches the gastric reservoir. Most of the organisms are killed by the hydrochloric acid present in the stomach (10^5 to 10^6 organisms per gram are killed in the stomach under normal conditions). The stomach is thus not only functional as an organ for proteolysis of ingested food; it is also a decontamination centre.

(3) The microbial barrier

Certain areas of the body are normally sterile, e.g. bladder, meninges, joints, the blood stream. The presence of bacteria in a site which is normally sterile constitutes an infection.

Certain areas of the body have a bacterial population. The anatomical areas which normally support a bacterial population include skin, vagina and the gastro-intestinal tract. An alteration in this normal population may predispose to disease by permitting superinfection of the area by various pathogens, e.g.:

(i) The intestine. Prolonged broad spectrum therapy leads to depletion of normal bowel flora. Superinfection by candida or pathogenic bacteria is thus facilitated. The mechanisms whereby the normal microbial bowel flora prevents the establishment of foreign or pathogenic organisms is not proven. Postulates include competition for nutrients, the establishment of a redox potential suitable for the normal commensal and not for the visitors, and also the production of various substances toxic to bacteria by strains different to that of the producer, e.g. colicines.

(ii) The vagina — in the post-menopausal female there is a change in the vaginal pH. The vagina becomes less acid and more susceptible to infection in the elderly female. In the menstruating female the hormonal balance dictates a high glycogen content in the superficial cells of the vagina. The normal microbial flora of the vagina includes lactobacilli. These organisms metabolize the glycogen converting it to lactic acid. The lactic acid produced decreases the vaginal pH creating an acid environment in the vagina of the menstruating female.

Table IV

THE ANATOMICAL DISTRIBUTION OF THE MICROBIAL BARRIER

STERILE ANATOMICAL AREAS

Fluids: blood
            cerebrospinal fluid

Serous cavities: pleura   nasal sinuses
                     peritoneum
                     meninges
                     joint cavities

Organs: All internal organs — muscle
                                   brain
                                   liver
                                   kidney
                                   heart
                                   bladder

ANATOMICAL AREAS WITH A BACTERIAL/MICROBIAL POPULATION
        Skin
        Mouth
        The respiratory tract
        Gastro-intestinal tract
        Vagina

Once the superficial defence barrier is breached the invader meets a secondary defence system.

(*b*)   SECOND LINE DEFENCE

This depends on the interaction between two defence components — cellular and humoral. The response of the host at this stage is aimed at handling any insult or injury to which it is exposed. It is non-specifically designed to help the host cope with a large variety of threats to its well-being.

Cellular Defence

The cellular defence at the level of non-specific immunity depends on the ability of certain cells to phagocytose organisms. The cellular systems responsible for phagocytosis are the polymorphonuclear leucocyte series and the mononuclear phagocytic cells.

This latter group includes fixed macrophages, and the circulating monocytes from which these are derived. Macrophages act as a link between innate and specific immunity.

The polymorphonuclear leucocyte matures in the bone marrow and is released into the blood stream. Neutrophils, basophils and eosinophils are found circulating in the blood. The neutrophil is the predominant species.

The mature neutrophil has certain abilities:
  (i) It is capable of moving to a specific site due to the release of certain chemicals at that site — chemotaxis.
 (ii) It is capable of phagocytosing particles — including organisms.
(iii) It is capable of digesting and/or killing ingested particles. This latter depends on the constituents of the particle ingested.

Eosinophils — these kill organisms about half as efficiently as neutrophils. Their numbers increase particularly in the presence of parasitic infections.

Basophils — these cells are pockets of vaso-active enzymes.

The process of phagocytosis

(*a*) *Adherence:* Contact between the organism (particle) and the cell membrane of the phagocyte is essential. Certain organisms/particles are inherently resistant to phagocytosis and the phagocyte may resort to certain tactics to overcome this —
  (i) Surface phagocytosis — it is easier for a phagocyte to ingest particles in rough confined areas, e.g. alveoli, than in wide open spaces, e.g. the peritoneum. The phagocyte 'corners' the organism.
 (ii) Opsonins — these may be specific antibody, non-specific immunoglobulin or protein products of the complement cascade. Both complement and antibodies have specific binding sites for receptors on cell membranes of phagocytes. Opsonins coat the organism facilitating adherence between the organism and the cell membrane. Bacteria and polymorphs each with a negative surface charge are mutually repulsive; neutralization of the organism's surface charge would decrease this. Opsonins may facilitate adherence by decreasing this electrostatic repulsion. Opsonins are particularly important in phagocytosis by the reticulo-endothelial (fixed macrophage) system.

Figure 2
PHAGOCYTOSIS

ADHERENCE

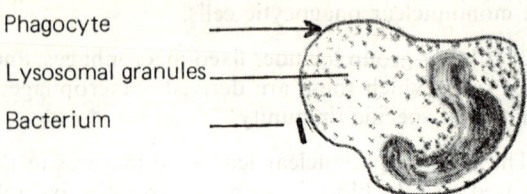

Phagocyte

Lysosomal granules

Bacterium

INGESTION

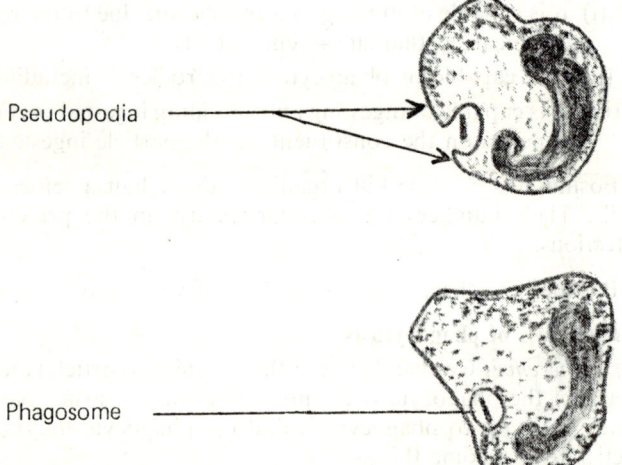

Pseudopodia

Phagosome

DIGESTION

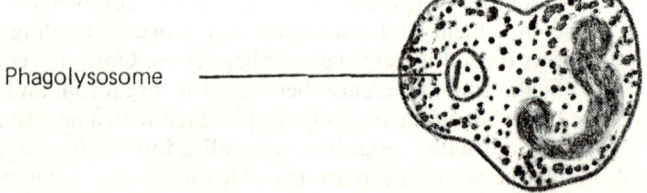

Phagolysosome

(*b*) *Ingestion:* The phagocyte extrudes pseudopodia (cytoplasmic protrusions) and surrounds the adhering organism with these cytoplasmic arms. The tips of the pseudopodia meet on the far side of the organism. The cell membrane in contact on the far side of the organism undergoes lysis and rejoins. The end result of this is a membrane bound organelle containing the organism. This is termed a phagosome. The phagosome is a membrane bound organelle containing the ingested particle/organism within the cell's cytoplasm.

Within the cytoplasm of phagocytes are membrane bound packets of hydrolytic enzymes — lysosomes. Fusion of the phagosome with one or more lysosomes results in the formation of a membrane bound phagolysosome.

(*c*) *Digestion:* Ideally once the organism lies within the phagolysosome it is subject to enzymatic digestion and death. The organism within the phagolysosome is exposed to enzymes capable of breaking down proteins, sugars, lipids and phospholipids. Various bactericidal substances, e.g. phagocytin and the myeloperoxidase — hydrogen peroxide — halogen (Cl, Br, I) system are also present. Errors in this system leading to leakage of lysosomal enzymes into the cells cytoplasm can result in host cell (phagocyte) death. Occasionally the organism resists digestion and uses the host cell as a transport vehicle and food factory.

The function of the cellular non-specific host defences is thus aimed at removal of particulate matter — including bacteria — from the extracellular environment. Once ingested the phagocytic cells attempt to catabolize the particle. The cell types involved are phagocytes; the mechanism is phagocytosis.

Humoral defences
Humoral defences are orientated towards facilitating host defences. They attempt to do this by:

(i) Aiding phagocytosis — both directly and indirectly.
(ii) Interacting with the specific humoral immune system in bringing about bacteriolysis.

The side effects of components of humoral non-specific immunity may have deleterious effects on the host. Inflammation leading to tissue injury is a reflection of harmful side effects associated with mechanisms used in defence of the host.

Components of non-specific humoral immunity include:
(i) *Opsonins* — these are antibodies which are found circulating at the time of the infection and are not specifically stimulated in response to this infection. These 'non-specific' antibodies may coat the invading organism and thus facilitate adherence between the phagocyte and the invading bacterium.
(ii) *Lysozyme* — this enzyme present in small amounts in tissue is iden-

tical to that found in various secretions including tears. It acts on the peptidoglycan layer of gram positive bacteria leading to a defective cell wall.

(iii) *Complement* — this system of proteins is found in normal serum. Activation of one component leads to activation of a second component and thus to a complement cascade. The complement cascade is reminiscent of blood coagulation in that the activation of one factor leads to the activation of the next factor in the series.

Complement may be directly activated by antigen/antibody reactions or indirectly by endotoxin. Endotoxin, present in all Gram-negative bacteria, activates complement via the alternate complement pathway.

Various activated components of complement have specific functions attributable to them. The overall effect of complement is to aid phagocytosis —

(i) *Directly* — adherence between bacteria and phagocytes is promoted. Immune adherence of organisms to cells facilitates surface phagocytosis.

(ii) *Indirectly* — leucocytes are chemically attracted to the area where complement has been activated. The phagocytes are thus chemotaxed to the vicinity of the bacterium.

Anaphylatoxin — this substance, by activation of histamine, leads to an increased blood flow to the area.

The nett effect of these components of complement is —

(i) to attract phagocytes to the site,

(ii) to facilitate phagocytosis by the phagocyte.

Complement reacting with specific antibody can result in lysis of Gram-negative bacteria. This is related to the interaction of complement and antibody on the lipopolysaccharide layer of the cell wall.

Many of the factors important in non-specific immunity are important in inflammation. Release of lysosomal enzymes from granulocytes into tissue, complement activation of kinens, and the blood clotting sequence are all systems poised to respond to any insult suffered by the host. The host's response to an organism at this level is similar to that towards an inert particle.

Inflammation measures the host's response to trauma; infection is inflammation associated with the presence of an organism. Inflammation is only part of the infection story. Infection need not be present for inflammation to occur; inflammation is present when infection occurs.

SUMMARY OF NON-SPECIFIC IMMUNITY

Superficial barrier: Mechanical
                             Chemical
                             Microbial

Aim — to prevent colonization and the establishment of organisms in anatomical sites usually free of those organisms.

Second line defences

(*a*) *Cellular* — Mechanism: Phagocytosis

Cell type: Polymorphonuclear leucocytes (circulate in the blood)

Mononuclear phagocytes (monocytes in the blood; macrophages in tissue).

Aim — digestion and killing of the organism.

(*b*) *Humoral* — Aid to phagocytosis — chemotaxis

opsonization

Cause defects in bacterial cell walls — Bacteria rendered more susceptible to the host's defences.

Aim — to elevate the host's resistance; to decrease bacterial pathogenicity.

Nett — A non-specific mechanism aimed at preventing colonization and multiplication of the foreign invader in the host is the host's immediate defence against the organism. The host depends on his non-specific defences to give him time to muster a response with weapons specifically adapted to cope with the invader. The macrophage is the main link between non-specific and specific immune factors. If the non-specific defences overcome the organism then stimulation of the specific immune mechanisms ceases; should the organism overwhelm the non-specific defences then the specific defences take up the battle. In such a case the non-specific defences join with the specific defences of the host in an attempt to overcome the invading organism. The examples of antibody acting as an opsonin and aiding phagocytosis and of antibody and complement lysing bacteria are both demonstrations of this co-operation.

B. SPECIFIC DEFENCES

The specific immune response has two arms — one cellular, the other humoral. Specific immunity depends on the ability of the body to recognise the organism as foreign. Certain biochemical sequences within the structure of the organism are different from those with which the host is acquainted. These biochemical sequences are called antigens. An antigen has certain properties:

(i) It is foreign to the host.

(ii) It illicits an immune response in the host. The immune response may be humoral, i.e. an antibody response; or cellular — a cell mediated response.

(iii) The antigen is capable of reacting with the immune response which is illicited, e.g. $Ag + Ab = AgAb$ reaction. The biochemical sequence of the antigen may be polypeptide, polysaccharide, alone or in various combinations with each other or with lipid.

It is postulated that the organism, with its antigenic constituents, is phagocytosed by a macrophage. The macrophage is thought to process the antigen and pass on this information to the lymphocyte series. Depending on the antigen involved the predominant stimulus will be directed either towards a humoral or cell mediated immune response.

Figure 3
SPECIFIC IMMUNITY

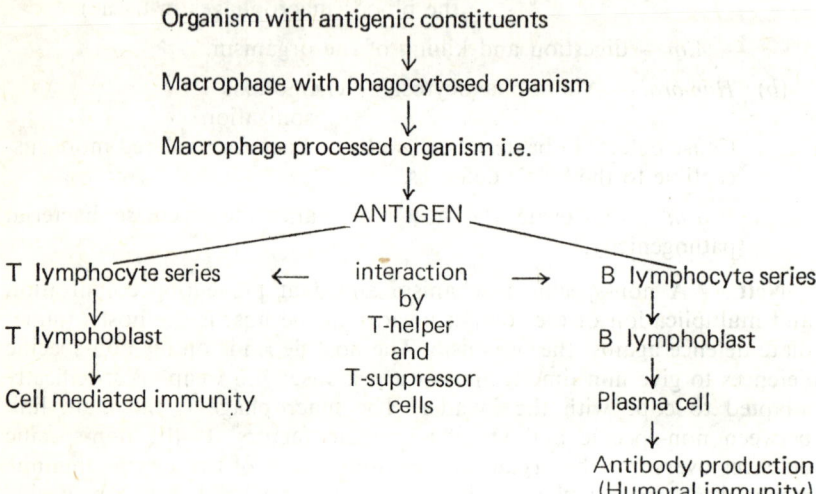

Organism with antigenic constituents
↓
Macrophage with phagocytosed organism
↓
Macrophage processed organism i.e.
↓
ANTIGEN

T lymphocyte series	←	interaction by T-helper and T-suppressor cells	→	B lymphocyte series
↓				↓
T lymphoblast				B lymphoblast
↓				↓
Cell mediated immunity				Plasma cell
				↓
				Antibody production (Humoral immunity)

(a) Humoral immunity

Specific humoral immunity is based on the production of antibodies. Antibody production depends on the B cell series. B lymphocytes have a short life span measured in days. B lymphocytes differentiate to form plasma cells. The plasma cell is directly responsible for antibody secretion. An antibody is a protein which is produced by the host in response to stimulation of his immune system by a foreign antigen. On electrophoresis antibodies migrate as globulins. Another name for antibodies is immunoglobulins (Ig). There are a number of classes of antibodies. Those important in protecting the host are —

> gamma globulin (IgG)
> meu globulins (IgM)
> alpha globulins (IgA)

IgG and IgM are serum antibodies, IgA is a secretory antibody. Antibodies produced in minute quantities include IgD and IgE. All these antibodies or immunoglobulins are produced by plasma cells.

Antibodies, like all proteins are composed of polypeptides. The basic unit of structure of an antibody is four polypeptide chains. Two of these chains are large and termed heavy chains; two are smaller and termed light chains. The body produces five different kinds of heavy chains —

α, γ, μ, δ, or ε. The type of heavy chain present in the antibody molecule determines the terminology of that molecule. There are two possible types of light chains — kappa or lambda. In any single antibody molecule there are two identical light chains and two identical heavy chains. The four chains are linked by disulphide bonds. A molecule of IgA contains two of these basic units, i.e. it contains a total of four light chains and four alpha chains. A molecule of IgM contains a combination of five of these basic units — ten light chains and ten meu chains.

Figure 4
THE STRUCTURE OF AN ANTIBODY

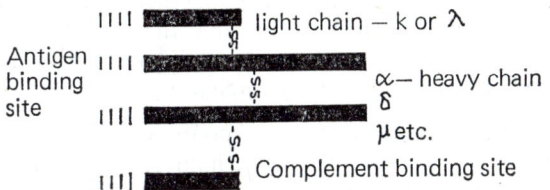

Each of these antibody units has along each of its chains an area which has a variable aminoacid sequence and an area which has a constant aminoacid sequence. The area of the constant aminoacid sequence on the heavy chain lies parallel to the area of the constant aminoacid sequence on the light chain. Complement attaches to a particular area of the constant aminoacid sequence of the antibody. It is this constant sequence of aminoacids which determines the characteristic features of the kappa or lambda light chain or the alpha or gamma heavy chain. The variable sequence of aminoacids is the area to which the antigen attaches. The area to which a particular antigen attaches is specific for that particular antigen. Two theories have been proposed to explain the formation of such a large variety of specific combination sites. The Instructive hypothesis suggests that the globulin formed is non-specific until such time as it contacts the macrophage processed antigen. The processed antigen then imposes upon the immunoglobulin the structural configuration which determines its antigenic specificity. The Selective theory suggests that each individual has within his genetic computor information on how to produce antibodies with specific binding sites for all possible antigens. This hypothesis claims that the macrophage processed antigen acts at the level of DNA and therefore the genetic code. It is suggested that repressed DNA is derepressed. Once functional this DNA directs protein synthesis by production of a mRNA template which produces antibodies specifically active against the stimulating antigen.

The function of antibodies

(i) To facilitate phagocytosis —

    (a) by agglutination and thereby immobilization of organisms;

(b) by opsonization of organisms and thereby facilitation of adherence between phagocyte and organism.

(ii) To kill bacteria — by interaction between complement and antibody. This leads to immune lysis of gram negative bacteria.

(iii) To neutralize secretory products of organisms, e.g. bacteria and render these non-toxic, i.e. antitoxin (antibody) can combine with toxins (antigen). This property of antibodies is the basis of immunization against a number of diseases, e.g. diphtheria, tetanus.

(iv) To prevent the first phase of infection by viruses. Antibody can interfere with the adsorption of viruses onto host cells.

Antibodies are found in the blood, the tissue fluid and also on all secretory surfaces. IgA antibodies thus form part of the superficial barrier on all mucous membranes. This once again illustrates that the immune response is the combined effort of a number of systems interacting in an attempt to protect the body against invasion by foreign organisms.

A primary response is the specific immune response which follows initial exposure to an antigen. In the case of specific humoral immunity a lapse of 2 to 3 weeks occurs between initial exposure to the antigen and the production of specific antibody. The antibody produced lasts for a limited period. The secondary immune response is the specific immune response of the host on second and subsequent exposures to the antigen (organism). In the case of humoral immunity the antibodies produced are produced far quicker — in a matter of days — and reach higher blood levels and are of a better quality. These antibodies remain at reasonably high levels within the blood for months after exposure to the antigen — the duration of antibody protection after a secondary immune response is of far longer duration than after a primary immune response.

If the individual is exposed to an antigen on more than two occasions his response is reminiscent of the secondary response. In vaccination schedules booster inoculations are given to maintain a high level of immunity.

(b) Cellular immunity

Intact cell mediated immunity is thought to be dependent on the presence of a normal thymus gland in intra-uterine life and early childhood. The T-lymphocyte series is the cellular unit involved. Once this series has been stimulated by processed antigen the cells differentiate into three functional types of cells:

(a) Memory cells
(b) Killer (cytotoxic) cells
(c) Helper and suppressor cells

T-cells have a long life — a lifespan measured in months.

The function of memory cells
Memory cells, as the name implies, are able to recall previous exposure to a particular antigen. When a memory cell contacts an antigen which it

recognises it immediately begins a series of differentiations into cells with cytotoxic or lymphokine functions. Memory cells shorten the time lapse between antigenic exposure and the specific host response. In the absence of specifically primed memory cells the time lapse between exposure and the specific cellular response is 10-14 days; in the presence of specifically primed memory cells this delay decreases to 48-72 hours.

Cytotoxic cells — these cells are poised to kill or remove any antigen to which they have been previously exposed (sensitised). These lymphocytes are a major problem in transplant surgery where the foreign antigen is the donor organ. Rejection is the expression of cell mediated immunity functioning in its normal capacity. The function of these cells is to eliminate foreign antigens.

Memory cells and cytotoxic cells are specific. This specificity is true both in terms of their response to stimulation and also in the expression of their function. Lymphokine producing cellular elements respond to a specific stimulus but the expression of their function is non-specific.

Lymphokines — this is the term used to encompass a large number of substances secreted by this series of T-lymphocytes. Lymphokines assist the host's immune response. The substances secreted are non-specific in their effect. Their action is not directed against a specific antigen; they are, however, stimulated to secrete their lymphokines on exposure to a specific antigen. The overall effect of lymphokines is to increase the host's ability to successfully eliminate any invading organism. Among the lymphokines are —

> *chemotactic factors* — chemical substances which attract phagocytes to the area of the antigen (organism)
> *macrophage inhibition factor* — MIF prevents the phagocytic monocytes from leaving the area

Figure 5
A SUMMARY OF SPECIFIC IMMUNITY

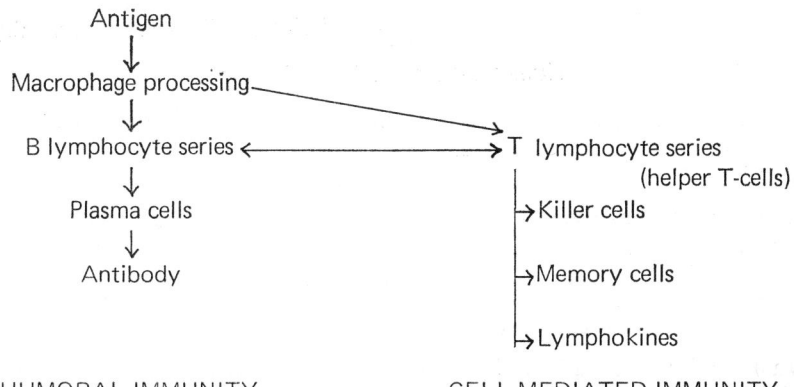

HUMORAL IMMUNITY   CELL MEDIATED IMMUNITY

> *macrophage activation factor* — MAF increases the metabolic acti-
> vity of the macrophages thereby supplying additional energy for
> phagocytosis and digestion of the foreign substance (organism)

Lymphokines thus conform to the other components of the immune system in that they are functionally orientated towards increasing the host's
efficiency in handling and eliminating foreign matter.

Specific immunity is geared to handle a number of foreign stimuli. It
has humoral and cellular branches — these interact and complement each
other. Cell mediated immunity is especially important in controlling and
eliminating those organisms capable of surviving and multiplying inside
cells. Humoral immunity is specialized in handling extracellular organisms.
Antibodies are orientated towards neutralizing toxins, assisting phagocytosis and preventing the adherence and hence the entry of viruses into
cells.

Figure 6
A SUMMARY OF HOST DEFENCES

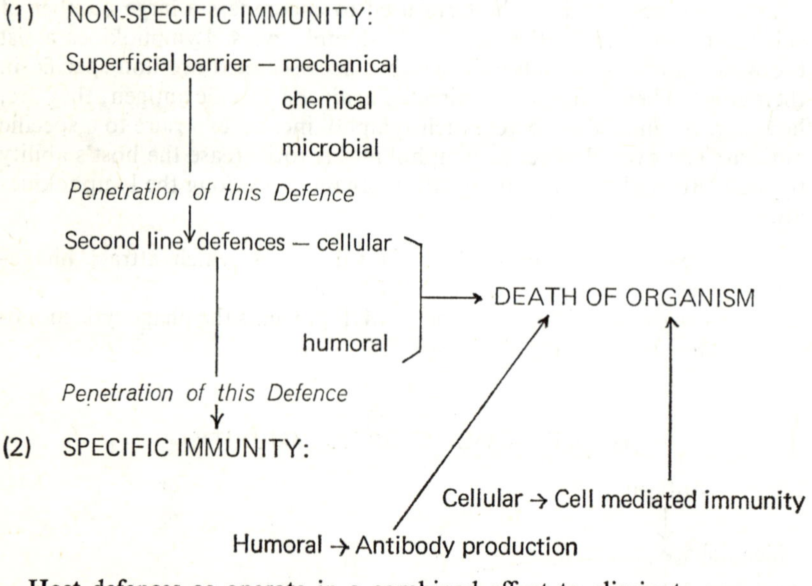

(1)   NON-SPECIFIC IMMUNITY:

Superficial barrier — mechanical
                      chemical
                      microbial

Penetration of this Defence

Second line defences — cellular

                                              ——→ DEATH OF ORGANISM

                        humoral

Penetration of this Defence

(2)   SPECIFIC IMMUNITY:

                              Cellular → Cell mediated immunity

Humoral → Antibody production

Host defences co-operate in a combined effort to eliminate any organism which may have established itself due to a defect in the superficial
barrier.

Some workers feel that the role of host defences is ultimately more
important than the virulence of the organism in determining the course
of many host-parasite relationships.

THE PARASITE / THE ORGANISM

In order for the parasite to become a pathogen it must overcome the host's
defences and cause disease in the host. A pathogen requires certain condi-

tions in the host and the environment, in addition to qualities within its own constitution in order to cause disease:

(*a*) The host must be susceptible — if the host has previously been exposed to the pathogen and his immune system is primed against the pathogen the chances of the pathogen establishing an infection in the host are extremely low. An immune host defends himself against the organism and kills it before it has an opportunity to gain a foothold. The organism is not given the opportunity to adapt itself to the host and to multiply.

The organism thus requires a host who has no specific immune response directed against it (the organism). Organisms not usually pathogenic can cause disease if the host's defences are defective, e.g. in the malnourished, the diabetic or the immunosuppressed. These people constitute a hyper-susceptible population.

(*b*) Factors contributing to pathogenicity — pathogenicity is the ability of the organism to cause disease; virulence is the degree of pathogenicity. A non-pathogenic organism or saprophytic organism lacks the factors necessary to cause disease.

Micro-organisms cause disease by —
(i) infection, i.e. invasion of, and multiplication in living tissue; and
(ii) via the production of pre-formed toxins which gain entry to the host via ingestion, inoculation or diffusion. This latter is a minor mechanism.

PATHOGENICITY

Infection depends on pathogenicity — the organism must spread to the new host and must multiply within the host. It may then impair both the structure and function of the host cell. Pathogenicity depends on communicability and virulence factors.

(1) COMMUNICABILITY

Communicability involves two concepts —
A. Transmissibility — the transfer of organisms to a new host
B. The Infective Dose — this is the number of organisms required to successfully colonize a new host

A. Transmissibility

Two factors greatly influence transmissibility:

(*a*) The anatomical site of the infection influences the possible routes of spread. A sneeze or cough may disperse respiratory pathogens; it will not disperse intestinal organisms.

(*b*) The resistance of the organism to environmental factors. Transfer of a large number of dead organisms to a new host is of no significance to either party. Certain organisms are capable of producing resistant spore forms in the presence of an unfavourable environment. Spores resist heat, cold, dessication and most chemical disinfectants. Sporulation is a protective and not a reproductive mechanism — spores survive but do not multiply. When conditions become favourable the spore form germinates reverting back to a vegetative, multiplying, pathogenic form of the organism. Spore forming organisms are found amongst the Clostridium genus — members of which cause tetanus, gas gangrene and botulism. Organisms not capable of forming spores display varying degrees of susceptibility to environmental conditions. All vegetative organisms are more susceptible to environmental factors than spores. Amongst the vegetative organisms more resistant to dessication are the staphylococci — they can survive for long periods in dust. Staphylococci are, however, susceptible to ultra-violet light and thus only survive under beds or in rooms from which sunlight has been excluded. *Neisseria gonorrhoeae*, the bacterium responsible for gonorrhoea is a very fastidious organism unable to resist adverse conditions. Especially fragile organisms are adapted to specialized modes of spread.

Many organisms are susceptible to drying, to temperatures above 60-65°C, to ultra-violet light and to chemicals.

Routes of Spread
Organisms spread from one host to another or from the environment to a host using different routes of spread. The route selected by a species is dependent on —

(*a*) the resistance of that organism to environmental factors
(*b*) the mechanism of spread available to that organism, and
(*c*) the portal of entry into the new host which is available to the organism.

Organisms may penetrate their new host's superficial defences by —

(*a*) ingestion
(*b*) inhalation
(*c*) transplacental spread
(*d*) penetration of the skin or mucous membranes by —
    (i) inoculation
    (ii) a defect in the physical barrier, e.g. due to trauma
    (iii) active penetration.

Organisms may spread by one of the following mechanisms —

(*a*) *Droplet spread* — coughing, sneezing and speaking are all associated with the spraying of individuals and objects in the immediate vicinity with a fine droplet spray. The droplet and organism, depending on particle size, may be immediately inhaled or settle on a surface. The larger particles settle while smaller particles remain airborne for variable distances. Once the droplets lose their moisture the resistance of the organism to dessication can determine whether the organism will remain viable or not.

The most difficult route of spread to eliminate in environmental control is droplet spread.

(*b*) *Contact* —

 (i) *Indirect contact* — utensils, clothing, articles and other objects, e.g. fomites. An individual with shigella dysentry may go to the toilet, contaminate his hands and then the door handle with bacilli. The door handle can then act as a vehicle in the transmission of infection. People touching the infected handle can transfer bacilli from the handle to their mouths via their hands. Shigella dysentry can be caused by as little as 10^4 organisms.

 (ii) *Direct contact* — person to person spread. A handshake may be an introduction to disease.

(*c*) *Venereal spread* — Organisms highly susceptible to environmental conditions are safely spread by sexual intercourse. Mucous membrane contact eliminates the problems of temperature change, drying and exposure to ultra-violet light. These problems are only experienced by organisms with a less sophisticated mode of transfer.

(*d*) *Arthropod borne disease* — Certain organisms undergo growth, multiplication and differentiation in an anthropod vector. Plasmodium, the parasite responsible for malaria, undergoes part of its life cycle in the mosquito. Arthropods may thus assist in the spread of disease in a variety of ways —

 (i) they may function as hosts during a stage of development of the organism

 (ii) they may act as vectors of disease — arthropods may be used as reservoirs for organisms, they may be instrumental in assisting the organism to penetrate the host's superficial barrier or they may merely act as mechanical vectors.

(*e*) *Congenital spread* — Certain organisms can cross the placenta and infect the foetus. These organisms are blood borne.

Table V

EXAMPLES OF IMPORTANT OR FREQUENTLY ENCOUNTERED
ORGANISMS ACCORDING TO THEIR PORTAL OF ENTRY

A. VIA INGESTION

Taenia	tape worms
Trichuris	whipworm
Enterobius	pinworm
Entamoeba	amoebiasis
Toxoplasma	toxoplasmosis
Clostridium botulinum	botulism
Salmonella	typhoid, gastroenteritis
Shigella	bacillary dysentry
Vibrio	cholera, foodpoisoning
Mycobacterium bovis	intestinal tuberculosis
Poliovirus	poliomyelitis
Coxsackievirus	pleurodynia, herpangina, aseptic meningitis
Echo	aseptic meningitis, febrile illness
Hepatitis A	infective hepatitis

Contamination of food, drink or eating utensils by any of the above organisms or their ova (in the case of the worms) can lead to infection via ingestion.

B. VIA INHALATION

Aspergillus	aspergillosis
Cryptococcus	cryptococcosis
Coccidiodes	coccidiodomycosis
Histoplasma	histoplasmosis
Streptococcus	sore throat, pneumonia
Neisseria	meningitis
Corynebacterium	diphtheria
Brucella	brucellosis
Haemophilus	meningitis, respiratory tract infection
Bordetella	whooping cough
Yersinia pestis	pneumonic plague
Mycobacterium	tuberculosis, leprosy
Mycoplasma	pneumonia
Coxiella	Q fever
Chlamydia	psittacosis
Herpes III	chicken-pox
Pox viruses	smallpox
Adenovirus	upper and lower respiratory tract infections
Rhinovirus	common cold
Influenzavirus	influenza
Parainfluenzavirus	laryngo-tracheo bronchitis, croup, upper and lower respiratory tract infections
Respiratory syncitial virus —	respiratory illness bronchiolitis ($<$6 month old)
Rubella	German measles
Rubeola	measles
Mumps virus	parotitis, orchitis

C. VIA PENETRATION OF THE SKIN

(i) Active Penetration —

Schistosomes	bilharzia
Ancylostoma, Necator	hookworms

(ii) Inoculation, e.g. via mosquito bites, tse-tse fly bites, etc.

Trypanosomes	sleeping sickness
Leishmania	cutaneous, muco cutaneous leishmaniasis, Kala-azar
Plasmodia	malaria
Yersinia pestis	bubonic plague
Borrelia	relapsing fever
Rickettsia	typhus node
Hepatitis B	serum hepatitis
Arboviruses	dengue, yellow fever

(iii) Via skin lesions, e.g. cuts, abrasions, etc.

Trypanosoma cruzi	Chagas disease
Epidermophyton, Trichonphyton, Microsporum	ringworm
Candida	candidosis
Sporothrix	sporotrichosis
Phialophora	chromomycosis
Staphylococcus	impetigo, folliculitis, furuncles
Streptococcus	cellulitis, erysepilas, impetigo
Bacillus anthracis	anthrax
Clostridia	gas gangrene, tetanus
Brucella	brucellosis

C. VIA PENETRATION OF THE SKIN (*Continued*)

Pseudomonas	septicaemia
Leptospira	leptospirosis
Treponema	syphilis, pinta, yaws
Hepatitis B	serum hepatitis

D. VIA MUCOUS MEMBRANE CONTACT

Trichomonas	vaginitis
Neisseria	gonorrhoea
Brucella	brucellosis
Treponema	syphilis
Chlamydia	trachoma, lympho-granuloma venereum
Herpes I, II, III	blisters, ulcers
Hepatitis B	serum hepatitis

B. The infective dose

The infective dose is the number of organisms required to successfully infect a new host. This number includes a safety margin to allow for those organisms which will be killed by the host before the infection is established. The infective dose varies for different pathogens. Important determinants of the size of the infective dose are:

  (i) the anatomical site of entry,

 (ii) the organism's resistance or susceptibility to host defences, and

(iii) the ease with which the organism can adapt and multiply in its new surroundings.

Figure 7
THE PHASES OF BACTERIAL GROWTH

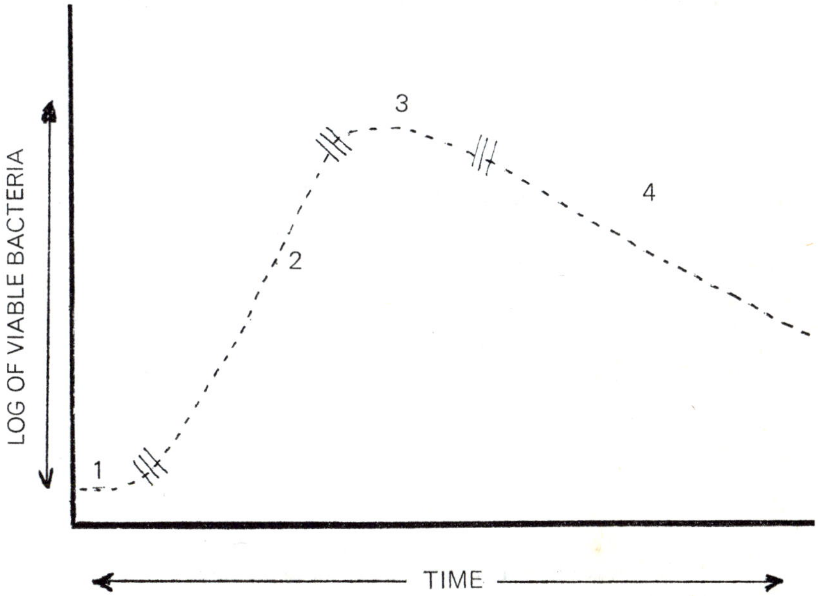

1 Lag phase.	2 Log phase.	3 Stationary phase.
4 Death phase	||| Transition periods.	

Bacteria in the log phase of growth are more likely to succeed in causing disease than organisms in the early lag phase of growth. An organism which is spread directly, e.g. venereal spread or droplet inhalation, has a better chance of being in the log phase of growth. The log phase of growth is that phase during which the organism rapidly undergoes multiplication (binary fission). There is a linear relationship between the log of the number of organisms and time. Organisms spread by indirect contact, e.g. dust are unlikely to be actively multiplying. They are more likely to be in a state of minimal growth, their energy being used in an attempt to survive the unfavourable environment. On introduction to a new host and more favourable environment, individual organisms start to increase their protein and enzyme synthesis. Bacteria in the lag phase are preparing themselves for a rapid multiplication spurt.

The infective dose of various bacteria differs — for *Yersinia pestis* the infective dose is one, for *Vibrio cholerae* it is 1×10^8. The infective dose and mode of spread are related, e.g. a low infective dose may be associated with direct or specialized spread, e.g. shigella dysentry spread by direct contact requires only 10 organisms to cause disease. Plague spread by the bite of an infected flea or droplet inhalation requires only one organism to cause disease. Organisms requiring a higher infective dose may require an opportunity to multiply on route, e.g. cholera organisms multiply in water and a high infective dose is required to cause disease as many bacterial lives are lost in the host's acid stomach; salmonella species multiply in food and reach the infective dose of 10^9 to 10^{11} organisms by using food as a culture medium. The infective dose is also related to the portal of entry. One hundred times more *Mycobacterium tuberculosis* organisms are required to infect the gastro-intestinal tract than the lung.

Table VI

AGENTS CAUSING EXOGENOUS AND ENDOGENOUS INFECTIONS

EXAMPLES OF ORGANISMS CAUSING EXOGENOUS INFECTIONS:

Worms pathogenic to man	
All organisms spread by vectors —	Trypanosomes
	Plasmodia
	Borrelia
	Yersinia
	Yellow fever
	Dengue
Virulent organisms	— Salmonella
	Shigella
	Entamoeba histolytica
	Rhabdovirus
	Hepatitis A and B virus

EXAMPLES OF ORGANISMS ASSOCIATED WITH ENDOGENOUS INFECTIONS:

Candida albicans	*Clostridium perfringens*
Actinomycetes	Herpes viruses
Escherichia coli	Bacteroides

When organisms are spread from the environment or from one host to another, then the infection is termed an Exogenous Infection. When the organism infecting an individual is derived from his own flora then the infection is termed an Endogenous Infection. Organisms which constitute part of the individual's normal flora only cause disease if they are —

(i) transferred from their usual site to a sterile area,

(ii) the host's defences become defective.

(2) VIRULENCE FACTORS

The success of the organism in invading host tissues depends on its ability to resist host defences. Host defences can be overcome by two basic mechanisms —

(*a*) the ability of the organism to resist death

(*b*) the organism's ability to cause disease in the host.

Of all micro-organisms it is bacterial virulence which has best been described. Many of the following remarks will thus refer to bacteria.

(a) The ability of the organism to resist death

(i) *The ability to resist cellular immunity*

The ability of the organism to resist death depends on its ability to resist cellular immunity, and this may be achieved by interference with phagocytosis —

(*a*) the ability to resist adherence and/or ingestion

(*b*) the ability to resist digestion

(*a*) *The ability to resist adherence and/or ingestion*

Surface infections occur via attachment of certain bacteria to epithelial cells, e.g. the K antigen of *E.coli* facilitates its attachment to intestinal mucous; *N.gonorrhoeae* attaches to the urethral mucosa via pili. The attached gonococcus is resistant to ingestion by phagocytes.

Organisms with capsules may depend for their pathogenicity on the presence of their capsule. *Streptococcus pneumoniae* resists phagocytosis due to the difficulty experienced by the polys in adhering to the organism. This organism is susceptible to digestion and thus can only multiply and cause disease outside cells. The host can overcome the defence of this organism by producing specific antibody. The antibody coats the organism making it susceptible to adherence and therefore ingestion. Other organisms which resist phagocytosis due to the presence of a capsule include *Haemophilus influenzae*, *Neisseria meningitidis*, *Yersinia pestis* and *Bacillus anthracis*.

(*b*) *The ability to resist digestion*

Certain organisms which are susceptible to adherence and ingestion may none the less be resistant to death once inside the phagocyte. They are able to resist digestion by the phagocyte. Organisms capable of resisting digestion by phagocytes find in their host cells a transport vehicle and a food factory. They are also protected by the cell from the host's extracellular defences.

Figure 8
A PICTORIAL DEMONSTRATION OF HOST PARASITE INTERACTION

E.g. Pneumococcal pneumonia

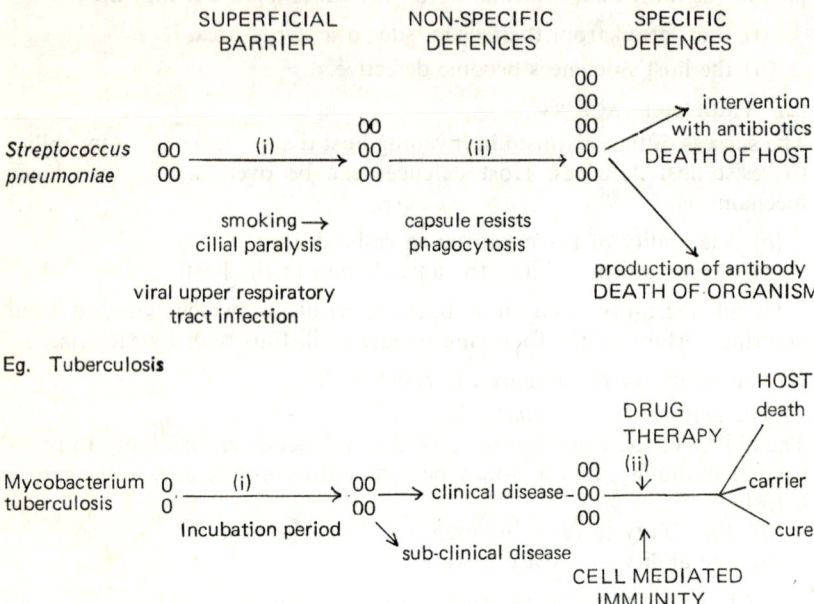

(i)   Multiplication of the organism
(ii) Infective individual — a danger to others —
      organism being shed.

Examples of groups of organisms capable of surviving intracellularly are the mycobacteria, fungi and viruses.

(ii) *The ability to resist humoral defences*

The K antigen of *E.coli* and the Vi antigen of salmonella are both capsular antigens capable of interfering with lysis of these gram negative organisms in the presence of complement. Humoral defences may fail to reach susceptible areas in the cell wall due to the protective effect of the acid polysaccharide component of these bacteria.

Viruses are obligate intracellular organisms. They evade the host's humoral immunity by —

(i) spreading directly from cell to adjacent cell. Antibodies neutralize viruses and prevent their penetration into cells;

(ii) latency — viruses can 'disappear' for variable periods. They then multiply, spread and cause disease when conditions are again favourable, e.g. the herpes group of viruses.

Certain organisms are capable of changing their antigenic structure, e.g.

borrelia, the spirochaete responsible for relapsing fever, and the trypanosomes are both thought to alter their surface characteristics so that the host's defences remain one step behind.

The above factors influence the ability of the organism to resist death. If the organism can remain viable and multiply it has the opportunity to produce various secretory products and toxins. These factors cause disease in the host and decrease the host's resistance. A decrease in host resistance gives the organism an opportunity to multiply and establish itself.

(b) The ability of the organism to cause disease

(*a*) *Secretion of enzymes:* A multitude of enzymes are secreted by different bacteria. Certain of these are thought to play a role in the pathogenesis of disease, e.g. hyaluronidase secreted by streptococci may play a role in the cellulitis associated with streptococcal infections; coagulase secreted by staphylococci may be one of the factors contributing to the localized boil characteristic of staphylococcal infections.

(*b*) *Secretions of toxins:* Toxins may initiate an infection, e.g. leucocidins may modify the clinical picture. Toxins may be the sole reason for the manifestations of a disease, e.g. tetanospasmin is responsible for the clinical picture of tetanus.

Toxins may have specific functions, e.g. leucocidins are toxic to white blood cells. The functions of certain toxins are common to a number of different bacteria, e.g. both staphylococci and streptococci produce leucocidins. Other toxins produce symptoms characteristic of certain organisms. Production of these toxins leads to the manifestation of specific clinical syndromes, e.g. *Clostridium tetani* releases a toxin which causes the clinical picture of tetanus; *Corynebacterium diphtheriae* releases its toxin and causes diphtheria. These latter toxins are not only highly specific, they are also highly potent. Collectively they may be termed exotoxins. Exotoxins are usually proteins and are secreted by viable bacteria. Both Gram-positive and Gram-negative organisms secrete exotoxin.

Endotoxin is part of the bacterial cell wall in Gram-negative bacteria. It is released on lysis of the bacterium. Endotoxin is composed of lipopolysaccharide and the lipid portion of the molecule is responsible for its toxicity. Patients with severe gram negative septicaemia may die of endotoxic shock.

Virulence may be enhanced by the rapid passage of the agent through a series of susceptible hosts (as in epidemics); attenuation may be achieved by passage of the agent through a series of unfavourable culture media.

SIGNS DUE TO THE PHYSICAL PRESENCE
OF THE ORGANISM

Organisms may cause disease due to their size and the anatomical site which they occupy. A single hydatid cyst can cause paralysis if located in the spinal cord, ascaris can pass unobserved until it migrates into the bile duct and causes obstructive jaundice. The signs and symptoms of crypto-coccal meningitis are mainly due to the pressure effects caused by the presence of the fungus on the brain.

Table VII

A SUMMARY OF THE ROLE PLAYED BY THE INFECTIOUS AGENT IN THE PATHOGENESIS OF DISEASE

(*a*) COMMUNICABILITY — transmissibility
infective dose

(*b*) VIRULENCE —

(1) Virulence in relation to bacterial infections
Resistance to the host's defences

(i) Resistance to phagocytosis at the levels of adherence and/or ingestion, digestion

(ii) Resistance to the effect of humoral defences

The ability to lower the host's defences

(i) Secretion of enzymes

(ii) Secretion of exotoxins

(iii) Release of endotoxin on lysis.

(2) Virulence in relation to viral infections

(i) The ability of the virus to convert the cell's machinery to a system whereby new virus is produced —
cells in many organs infected
cells of target organs infected

(ii) Spread of virus to uninfected cells by continuity and contiguity

(iii) Latency.

(3) Virulence in relation to protozoan and other parasitic infections.
The virulence factors in these cases are variable and often poorly described.

THE HOST RESPONSE

The response of the host to the presence of foreign material in the body is an attempt to eliminate the foreign organism. The manner in which the host attempts to achieve this is not without cost. The immune response as well as the inflammatory response have both beneficial and harmful components. An exaggerated attempt to get rid of the organism can result in harmful consequences, e.g. the caseation and fibrosis associated with a tuberculous lung infection may be of value in attempting to rid the host of the mycobacterium, it does also, however, result in irreparable loss of lung tissue. The chlamydia responsible for lymphogranuloma venereum and the microfilaria responsible for elephantiasis both illicit an exaggerated response in the host leading to excessive fibrosis with oedema. Even when the host is succeeding in lysing a large number of bacilli he may precipitate side-effects depending on his antibody level, e.g. erythema nodosum leprosum.

Once the organism has succeeded in infecting a new host it may be killed by the host or it may multiply and establish itself in the host. Certain diseases are characteristically associated with infection of man, e.g. gonorrhoea, whooping cough. Other organisms cause disease in animals and these organisms may then be transmitted to man. Diseases transmitted between animals and man are termed zoonoses. Once man has been infected the organism may be incapable of being transmitted to another host, e.g. sindbis is an end stage viral infection in man. Certain zoonoses may be transmitted further either directly, e.g. pneumonic plague, or indirectly by arthropod vectors, e.g. yellow fever. The transmission of endemic murine typhus, a rickettsial disease, is by the flea from rat to man; once man is infected further transmission to other humans is by the louse.

CONCLUDING REMARKS

The balance obtained between the host and the organism is expressed in the following situations:

Clinical or overt disease

In this case the pathogen has overwhelmed the host's defences and has multiplied in the host and caused disease. Bacillary dysentry, tetanus, rabies are all examples of clinically overt disease. The patient admitted to hospital is suffering from clinical disease.

Sub-clinical infection

In this case a balance between host and parasite has occurred. The balance is slightly in favour of the parasite allowing multiplication of the organism. The number of organisms produced or the virulence of these organisms is, however, insufficient to in any way cause the host overt inconvenience. Cholera is recognised as a disease with a large number of sub-clinical cases. Apparently healthy people with a positive tuberculin test are thought to house a viable and possibly multiplying mycobacterium. In cases with sub-clinical infection one may isolate the organism from the apparently healthy host under suitable conditions.

Latent infections

Sub-clinical infections are usually of short duration while latent infections may last a life time. In cases of latent infection it is often not possible to isolate the organism. Latent infection follows a period during which the patient has had apparent cure following a clinical or sub-clinical infection. During this latent period the organism appears to have been eliminated by the host's defences. Infection by this organism can again become overt should some stimulus alter the immune status of the host. Herpes hominis or Herpes type I causes gingivo-stomatitis, a primary overt clinical infection. The individual recovers and years later may present with fever blisters. The factor precipitating this relapse may be excess exposure to sunlight or an attack of pneumococcal pneumonia. Herpes type III causes chicken pox on primary exposure, in the older patient shingles may develop as a result of reactivation of the latent virus. Most people have immunity against cytomegalovirus as a result of latent infection; if this individual receives immunosuppressive therapy he may die from generalized cytomegalovirus infection.

The carrier state

An individual who is colonized by a pathogenic bacterium and is in good health is termed a carrier. The organism may be 'carried' by the host for a variable period of time, e.g. if an individual excretes *Salmonella typhi* for a three month period then the individual is termed an acute carrier; if he excretes *Salmonella typhi* for over one year then he is termed a chronic carrier.

The mode of acquisition of the organism may further help to classify the carrier state —

 (i) *Convalescent carriers* — these are patients who have recovered from their illness but are still secreting the organism.

 (ii) *Contact carriers* — in this case the individual secreting the organism has at no stage suffered from an illness caused by the organism. He has been in contact with a patient suffering from an infection caused by the organism.

 (iii) *Paradoxical carriers* — the organism is isolated from a healthy person who to his knowledge has had no contact with a patient suffering from the disease.

 (iv) *Intermittent carrier* — a healthy individual who may over a period alternate between being free of the organism and carrying the organism.

The carrier state is one in which the host and the pathogen have adapted to each other and are existing in a perfect balance.

Table VIII
PATHOGENS WHICH MAY BE ISOLATED FROM HEALTHY CARRIERS

Corynebacterium diphtheriae
Haemophilus influenzae
Streptococcus pneumoniae
Salmonella typhi
Vibrio cholerae
Neisseria meningititis
Staphylococcus aureus
Poliovirus
Coxsackievirus

SPREAD OF INFECTION IN THE HOST
Infection can be spread by the following routes —

 (i) *Continuity* — from cell to cell.

 (ii) *Contiguity* — along natural passages, e.g. infection of the tonsil can seed organisms into the respiratory tract.

 (iii) *Lymphatic spread* — the organism can drain from an area by the lymphatics. It is then either caught up in the lymph node filter, or passes into the blood stream via the thoracic duct. Lymphatic spread can also be retrograde, e.g. if a lymph node proximal to the lymphatic is blocked then the lymph will drain distal to the blocked area.

 (iv) *The blood stream* — Bacteraemia is associated with the temporary presence of bacteria in the blood stream; viraemia with the presence of viruses. Septicaemia is associated with the more prolonged presence of multiplying organisms in the blood stream. Bacteraemia may be transient and harmless, septicaemia is always associated with disease.

POSSIBLE OUTCOME OF INFECTION

(i) Death and elimination of the pathogen may result. The host may develop long lasting immunity against this species.

(ii) The pathogen may be localized as a boil.

(iii) The pathogen may spread — locally, e.g. cellulitis; by lymphatics e.g. lymphadenitis, lymphangitis; by blood, e.g. septicaemia.

(iv) A generalized disease may result — due to toxins, e.g. botulism — due to spread of the organism, e.g. miliary tuberculosis.

(v) Latency may develop.

Organisms may have local plus general effects. The local effects are associated with local interference with tissue function and metabolism. The pain, redness and swelling associated with inflammation may resolve or progress to permanent loss of normal function, fibrosis and scarring. Specialized tissue may regenerate or be permanently lost. Generalized effects vary for different organisms, e.g. most organisms induce fever in the host; diphtheria toxin interferes with the synthesis of proteins in distant target organs, tetanospasmin causes generalized spasms.

IMMUNITY

Immunity is the host's ability to evoke an immune response. It is his ability to defend himself against a specific insult (organism). On second and subsequent exposure to the organism his defences react more quickly and with greater strength. His response is enhanced both in terms of quantity and quality.

NATURAL IMMUNITY

This depends on non-specific host defences. A lowering of these defences can result in an increased susceptibility to infection. Malnourished individuals are at risk of acquiring the organism and also of developing a more severe infection. Measles in a malnourished individual is more frequently complicated by bronchopneumonia and otitis media. Measles is often fatal in the malnourished child, i.e. in the child with impaired natural defences against infection.

Natural immunity to certain diseases is related to an individual's genetic complement. Tuberculosis may be more prevalent in black than white races due to genetic differences between the races. Individuals with the sickle cell trait are resistant to *Plasmodium falciparum* malaria.

ACQUIRED IMMUNITY

This depends on the specific immune defences:

(a) *Passive immunity:* Passive immunity can be achieved in two ways —

by transplacental spread of antibody (materno-foetal transfusion); by intravenous infusion of antibody — hyperimmune serum may be used. Passive immunity is of limited duration.

(b) *Active immunity:* This is due to exposure of the individual's immune system to that particular antigen. The individual's immune system responds with stimulation of the appropriate defence system, i.e. by antibody production, by cell mediated immunity or both. A delay between first exposure to the antigen and the production of specific immunity occurs. This delay is shorter on subsequent exposure. Active immunity is of longer duration than passive immunity. The duration of active immunity may be further modified by the type of infecting organism. Immunity to whooping cough, diphtheria, smallpox or mumps is usually accepted as longer lasting than immunity to influenza. The shorter lasting immunity to influenza is mainly due to the organism's ability to alter its antigenic structure and therefore reappear as 'foreign' to the immune system. A further factor which may modify the duration of the host's immunity is that active immunity acquired as a result of infection of a mucosal surface appears to be of shorter duration than immunity acquired as a result of systemic infection.

SPECIFIC IMMUNITY AND HYPERSENSITIVITY

Both the cell mediated and the humoral arms of cell mediated immunity can ricochet and instead of protecting the host can damage the host. Specific immunity in most circumstances defends the host and is beneficial to the host. Should the host's immune system be defective and fail to react then the host becomes susceptible to his environment; should the immune system react in too vigorous a manner or in an abnormal manner hypersensitivity disease may result.

Humoral immunity is implicated in the following hypersensitivity reactions:

Type I

Reagenic hypersensitivity depends on the presence of reagin or IgE. This immunoglobulin is bound to mast cells. On exposure to the antigen an antibody-antigen reaction occurs on the surface of the mast cell. This results in the release of vasoactive substances from the mast cell. The release of histamine, kinins, serotonin and slow reactive substance affects the smooth muscle cells of arterioles and bronchioles. The effects of Type I hypersensitivity can be seen locally as bronchospasm, e.g. asthma, or systematically as the anaphylactic reaction where shock and vasodilation supervene.

Type II

Cytotoxic hypersensitivity. In this form of hypersensitivity the antibody binds to cells of the host. The antibody binds to host cells because the antigen with which the antibody specifically reacts is already attached to the cell. In measles a haemorrhagic diathesis may develop as the measles virus may in certain cases become attached to platelets. The host's antibody has been produced against the virus and thus the antibody attaches to infected platelets. The platelets with their antibody-antigen complex may then be phagocytosed or lysed should complement be fixed. The end result is a decrease in the number of platelets available in the circulation. The patient with an adequate platelet count is in danger of being unable to adequately control haemostasis.

Type III
Immune complex disease. Here immune complexes are formed which differ from the usual complex in that these complexes are formed in the presence of antigen excess and therefore fail to precipitate. The soluble complexes, unlike the larger precipitating complexes, are not taken up by the reticulo-endothelial system. The soluble and small complexes can be trapped in the small blood vessels of, e.g. the skin, causing skin rashes; the glomeruli of the kidney, causing glomerulonephritis; and the joints, causing arthritis. Inflammation in these sites occurs as a result of complement fixation by the immune complexes. Polymorphonuclear leucocytes are then attracted to the area. Examples of diseases in which immune complexes are believed to be the cause of the underlying pathology include rheumatoid arthritis, lupus erthematosis and erythema nodosum leprosum. Historically the example of localized immune complex disease is the Arthus reaction; the example of generalized immune complex disease is serum sickness.

Cell mediated immunity is also capable of causing harm to the individual:

Type IV
In Type IV hypersensitivity cell mediated immunity expresses itself with the harmful side effects of delayed hypersensitivity. Examples of delayed hypersensitivity are the caseous reaction which results in lung tissue destruction in pulmonary tuberculosis; contact dermitis is a frequently encountered form of delayed hypersensitivity.

Type V
Antibody may stimulate endocrine cells by acting on surface receptors.

Table IX
HYPERSENSITIVITY

TYPE	I Anaphylactic	II Cytotoxic	III Immune Complex Disease	IV Delayed Hypersensitivity	V Stimulatory
HOST RESPONSE MEDIATED BY:	Ige	Ig- + Complement	Ig- + Complement	T-lymphocyte	Ig
ANTIGEN	Exogenous	Cell surface	Extra-cellular	Variable	? Cell surface
EXAMPLE	Asthma anaphylaxis	Haemolytic anaemia e.g. sedormid	Immune nephritis	Tuberculin test	Thyrotoxicosis e.g. LATS

Both humoral and cellular immunity may be deficient and result in an inadequate response on exposure to antigens. The inability of the individual to mount an adequate immune response may be a congenital or an acquired defect. Congenital lack of immunoglobulins is associated with repeated bacterial infections. Congenital absence of the thymus results in defects of the cell mediated arm of immunity. Defective cell mediated immunity may only become apparent when the child is vaccinated against smallpox. Smallpox inoculation is fatal in children who lack cell mediated immunity. Certain diseases may depress cell mediated immunity, e.g. measles, Hodgkin's, metastatic tuberculosis, sarcoidosis and immuno-suppressive therapy. Defects of cell mediated immunity lead to suscepti-bility to fungi, pox and herpes viruses, and to infection by intracellular bacteria, e.g. mycobacteria (tuberculosis, leprosy), salmonella and brucella.

SEROLOGY

Serology is the diagnostic tool used in the detection and identification of disease by examination of the host's specific humoral response. Exposure of the individual to a specific organism usually results in production of antibodies. Antibodies so produced recognise and react with that orga-nism. Serology thus involves the use of laboratory techniques to detect the presence and quantity of antibody in the patient's blood.

Examples of laboratory techniques used include:

(a)   The precipitin test

(i) Antibody and colloidal antigen may be mixed in a test tube and allowed to form a lattice work. This forms at the optimal ratio.

(ii) Antibody and colloidal antigen may also be pipetted separately into agar wells and allowed to diffuse through the agar towards each other. Precipitation of antibody-antigen complexes will occur in the region of the agar gel where the antibody and antigen are in an optimal ratio.

In the area where there is either an excess of antibody or antigen the lattice formed is defective and not visible to the naked eye.

(b)   Agglutination tests

These resemble precipitation tests except that they are not done in an agar gel but only in the test tube. The antigen is particulate and the reaction between antibody and antigen is thus flocculant rather than granular.

(c)   Complement fixation tests

These depend on the principle that during certain antibody antigen reac-tions complement is fixed. A system involving the use of known antigen and unknown antibody is mixed and given an opportunity to interact. This system is then exposed to sensitized red blood cells. If complement is pre-sent, i.e. has not been used up by interaction between the unknown anti-body and known antigen, then the red blood cells will lyse (burst). In cases where the erythrocytes lyse the patient has not produced antibodies to the antigen (organism) being tested. When the erythrocytes remain intact there has been interaction between the known antigen and unknown antibody.

(d) Fluorescence tests

A fluorescent dye is attached to either a known antigen or a known antibody, this is then reacted with an unknown. If there is an antigen antibody reaction the fluorescence will remain attached to the unknown and this can thus be identified.

The basic principle involved is that the interaction between an antibody and an antigen is specific. Interaction between a known antigen with an unknown antibody leads to identification of the antibody and vice versa.

Estimation of the quantity of the antibody in the patient's serum is done by diluting the serum a certain number of times and testing the dilution against a constant quantity of antigen. The higher the dilution of serum capable of reacting with the antigen, the higher the concentration of antibody in the patient's serum. A rising titre means that the patient's serum when first taken reacted at a certain dilution with a certain quantity of antigen; when taken some time (2 weeks) later the antibody level had increased and a higher dilution of serum was then capable of reacting with the antigen and forming a reaction visible to the naked eye.

Serology is used both as an epidemiological tool and in the retrospective diagnosis of disease. When used as an epidemiological tool serology involves testing the host's blood to see if he has produced an immune response against a certain organism. The presence of antibodies in the blood of the individual implies that the individual has been exposed to the organism and is resistant to disease induced by that organism.

Serology is of value in —

(i) assessing the immune status of population groups

(ii) determining the susceptibility of populations to epidemics caused by certain virulent organisms

(iii) the retrospective identification of epidemics in terms of both the organism involved and the approximate year in which the last epidemic occurred.

In South Africa the secular trend of plague in the plague endemic areas has been determined by serology.

When serology is used in the retrospective diagnosis of disease a blood sample is tested for the presence of antibodies at the acute phase of the illness and a second blood sample is tested during the patient's convalescence. If there has been a four-fold rise in the antibody titre against a certain organism this is diagnostic of the patient's recent acute infection having been caused by this organism. Retrospective diagnosis does not help in the treatment of the patient but it does give the doctor an indication of which organisms are prevalent during a particular period. Patients are also much happier when they can tell their friends that they had a very bad attack of such and such. They like a definitive diagnosis to better clarify future discussions of their ailments.

PROBLEMS IN THE INTERPRETATION OF SEROLOGICAL RESULTS

Certain organisms have similar antigenic determinants, e.g. proteus and rickettsia have cross reacting antigens. If an individual who has previously had tick bite fever develops a urinary tract infection caused by a specific type of proteus his antibodies against *Rickettsia conori* will increase. This rise in antibody titre is due to his urinary tract infection and not due to tick bite fever. Syphilis may be provisionally diagnosed using certain screening tests. False positive results may be obtained if the individual is suffering from overt or subclinical measles, malaria, leprosy, is pregnant or has a collagen disease. An anamnestic response is the increase of antibodies in the patient's serum when that individual is not suffering from the disease suggested but from infection by an antigenically related organism. When an anamnestic response occurs the rise in antibody titre is always lower than in true infections by the organism. The rise in titre should be at least four-fold in cases of infection.

A single antibody test can be misleading as the individual may have antibodies as a result of inoculation or due to previous infections. In order to diagnose a recent acute infection the single antibody level must be extremely high or preferably a rising titre should be demonstrated.

Serology is a limited tool in the diagnosis of acute infection due to —
   (i) the persistence of serum antibody levels for long periods
   (ii) the delay in antibody production on primary exposure to an organism.

Table X

SOME DISEASES DIAGNOSED ON SEROLOGY

Syphilis
Typhoid
Brucellosis
Rickettsial diseases
Infectious mononucleosis

SKIN TESTS

These tests may be employed to test whether an immune competent host has been previously exposed to an organism or toxin. The more commonly used skin tests test the cell mediated immune system.

Skin tests used to diagnose previous exposure, infection and resistance dependent on the individual's cell mediated immune system include:
   (*a*) Tuberculin test
   (*b*) Candida skin test
   (*c*) Histoplasmin test
   (*d*) Lepromin test
   (*e*) Brucellin skin test

A suspension of the particular antigen is injected intradermally and the memory cells of the cell mediated immune system will set the wheels of cell mediated immunity in progress provided they recognise the antigen. The memory cells will only recognise the antigen if the individual has been previously exposed to the antigen, i.e. if the individual has been infected by the organism or immunized against the disease. In cases where the memory cells recognise the antigen a skin reaction develops within 48-72 hours at the site of infection. A positive skin reaction within this time period is interpreted as evidence that the individual has been previously exposed to the antigen (organism) and that the body has already learned how to handle the organism. The positivity of the skin test is probably not a reflection of the host's immunity but rather expressed the host's hypersensitivity response to that organism. A highly positive tuberculin skin test is suggestive of active disease requiring treatment; a moderately positive test is indicative of some immunity to the organism. A negative skin test indicates no immunity against this organism. In the case of the tuberculin skin test false positive results may be obtained if the individual has been infected by one of the mycobacteria other than tubercle bacilli (Mott bacilli). The genus *Mycobacterium* shares certain common antigens. The positivity of the skin test and the use of different inocula prepared from the previous mycobacteria can be used to overcome this difficulty.

A negative skin test may be interpreted in one of two ways:

(i) The test is truly negative and the individual has never been exposed to the organism, has no resistance to the organism and is a susceptible host. Inoculation to stimulate resistance against infection and disease by this organism may, in certain cases, be advised.

(ii) A false negative test. False negative tests may be obtained if the host has a defect in his defences, e.g. the immunosuppressed patient. False negative results in patients suffering from tuberculosis may be obtained on tuberculin testing in patients suffering from:

(*a*) malnutrition

(*b*) measles

(*c*) Hodgkin's disease

(*d*) sarcoidosis, or

(*e*) an overwhelming tuberculosis infection.

If an individual is tuberculin tested within 2 weeks of exposure and infection by *M.tuberculosis*, the skin test will also give a negative result. Tuberculin tests differ in the purity of the antigen used. Both the Heaf and the Mantoux tests are tests for tuberculosis.

Tests depending on the host's humoral immune response are seldom used today. Two tests are still worthy of mention.

The Dick Test — Erythrogenic toxin produced by *Streptococcus pyogenes* is injected into the forearm of the individual. If the injected area develops erythrema then the individual has no neutralizing antibodies present. This individual is susceptible to scarlet fever. An individual who has previously had scarlet fever has developed antibodies capable of neutralizing erythrogenic toxin. Such an immune individual does not develop a reaction at the injection site.

The Schick Test — This test is of value in differentiating between those susceptible to, and those resistant against diphtheria. The Schick test is still occasionally used to differentiate between susceptible and resistant members of the nursing staff.

Diphtheria toxin is injected into the forearm of the individual. The presence of specific antibody in the individual's blood will prevent a reaction developing. If the individual has not been immunized against, or been exposed to diphtheria a skin reaction will occur. A positive Schick reaction in a member of the nursing staff is an indication for immunization against diphtheria. A control inactivated heated toxin is always introduced into the opposite forearm to enable the person reading the test to differentiate between a true positive result and a hypersensitivity reaction to the injected material.

CHAPTER 3

The Laboratory Diagnosis of Disease

THE COLLECTION OF SPECIMENS

WHICH SPECIMEN SHOULD BE COLLECTED?

In certain cases a knowledge of the life cycle of certain parasites is necessary, in others it is sufficient to collect a specimen from the site inferred by the patient's signs and symptoms.

Chest pain plus a productive cough would point to a chest infection and sputum would be the obvious choice of specimen. Burning on micturition would point to a urinary tract infection and the specimen required is thus urine. If the condition of the patient in either case is critical septicaemia would be suspected and a blood culture may be performed.

THE LABEL

Correct labelling of a specimen is one of the most important tasks in the laboratory diagnosis of disease. The patient's name, ward and hospital number will lead to the patient getting a result on his own specimen. The specimen being submitted should be accompanied by information on the suspected diagnosis, the anatomical site from which the specimen was obtained and the investigations which the doctor wishes to be performed on the specimen. The name of the hospital from which the specimen is sent should also appear on the label.

HOW TO COLLECT SPECIMENS

Specimens which are submitted for microbiological investigation must:

(a) not be collected in formalin, alcohol or any disinfectant if culture or propagation of the organism is desired;

(b) not, in most cases, experience a delay of more than 60-90 minutes between collection and submission to the laboratory;

(c) be collected in a sterile container; and

(d) be collected taking care to avoid contamination of the specimen by microbial flora of the patient and environment, and also to avoid spread to others of a potentially harmful organism.

Sputum collection

The oropharynx has a normal flora. Bacteria are not normally found in the alveoli. When one is taking a sputum specimen two points must be remembered.

(i) The specimen must be a deep cough specimen — the bacteriologist is looking for the organism present in the bronchioles and the alveoli, not in the saliva. An early morning cough specimen is recommended. The sputum produced by the patient should be collected directly in the bottle supplied by the laboratory.

(ii) The specimen is going to be contaminated en route during its transfer from lung to oral cavity. The bacteriologist must therefore attempt to differentiate between normal flora of the upper respiratory tract and the organism causing the disease.

Sputum is at best a difficult specimen for the laboratory to correctly interpret. It is thus of great importance that the ward should submit a deep cough sputum specimen. Excessive delay between collection and laboratory processing of the specimen will further complicate interpretation of the cultural findings.

Urine collection

The bladder is a normally sterile area. In theory any organism found in urine could thus be termed a pathogen. In practise the method of urine collection alters laboratory findings. Urine runs from a sterile bladder, through the urethra, the distal portion of which is contaminated, and is then collected in a sterile receptacle. In the female this problem is magnified as the urethral orifice lies in the vulva, an area with a normal microbial flora.

There are certain basic precautions necessary in the collection of urine specimens.

(*a*) A midstream specimen must be collected. The patient is asked to void in stages. The portion of the urine first voided is used as a lavage for the urethra. The portion of the urine used to wash out the urethra is discarded. The next portion of the urine voided is collected in a sterile specimen bottle and submitted to the laboratory. The remaining urine is voided in the pan.

(*b*) A clean catch specimen is required. A mid-stream specimen will only constitute a clean catch if the following precautions are observed. In the male the prepuce and terminal portion of the penis must be thoroughly cleaned. In the female the vulval and perineal area should be swabbed. A vaginal plug should be inserted. Vaginal discharge contaminating a urine specimen will lead to a false result.

In spite of these precautions, bacterial contamination of urine specimens does occur and figures based on the probable significance of certain numbers of bacteria have been calculated.

Bacterial growth of less than 10 000 organisms per millilitre of urine is interpreted as probable contamination of the specimen; bacterial growth of more than 100 000 organisms per millilitre is interpreted as infection. Growth between 10 000 and 100 000 organisms per ml falls into a grey zone and further specimens should be submitted. Patients who are already catheterized should have catheter specimens submitted. The urine should be aspirated from the rubber tubing near to the catheter urine-bag connection. The area of the catheter selected for puncture should be disinfected prior to aspiration. Urine from the urine bag should not be submitted for investigation. The catheter and urine bag should not be disconnected in order to collect urine from the bladder. Catheterization in order to obtain a urine specimen is contra-indicated. In selected cases urine may be obtained by supra-pubic puncture.

The white cell count of urine is also of some value in the diagnosis of urinary tract infection. A count of over 4 000 white blood cells (polys) per millilitre is suggestive of infection.

Cerebrospinal fluid collection

Cerebrospinal fluid (CSF) is obtained by insertion of a needle into the spinal canal and drainage of fluid surrounding the brain and spinal cord. This fluid is normally sterile. The isolation of an organism from CSF is thus diagnostic provided the specimen is not contaminated during lumbar puncture. Contamination is avoided by adequate preparation of the patient's skin prior to insertion of the needle and by preparation of the operator as for a sterile procedure. CSF containing bacteria and white blood cells is indicative of meningitis.

Swabs

A dry swab of a dry lesion is of next to no value. A swab which reaches the laboratory after a 2 hour delay is of increasingly little value.

Swabs are often taken from anatomical sites which have a normal flora—it is thus vitally important that the site which has been swabbed be noted on the swab's label. Knowledge of the normal flora or the site swabbed may radically alter the laboratory interpretation of the organisms cultured. When swabbing an area, the most inflamed, most pussy area should be selected. When swabbing a skin lesion swab under a scab. Vesicles, abscesses and other fluid collections should, where possible, be aspirated rather than swabbed. Aspirates provide a larger quantity of the specimen, they also supply a specimen less likely to be contaminated by skin or environmental organisms.

Faecal specimens

Faeces contain of the order of 1×10^{14} organisms per gram (wet weight). The laboratory adapts to this bacterial load by culturing specimens on selective media. If a faecal specimen experiences a delay between collection and culturing the non-pathogenic bacteria normally present in faeces may overgrow the pathogens. False negative cultures may thus be due to a delay in the specimen reaching the laboratory. The quantity of stool submitted should be between 0,3 and 2,0 grams. Portions submitted should be selected, e.g. a mucus or blood stained sample may be submitted. At least three specimens should be submitted if the clinical picture is suggestive and the laboratory fails to isolate a pathogen.

Examination for amoebae should be done on a warm stool.

Blood

Blood is a sterile fluid. The presence of organisms in a blood culture means either that organism is present in the patient's blood or that contamination has occurred. Blood cultures should be collected using strict precautions. The patient's arm is prepared using both 70% alcohol and iodine prior to venepuncture. The individual doing the venepuncture should mask and scrub thoroughly. As bacteraemias can be intermittant it is necessary to take at least three blood cultures at intervals of at least one hour over a 24 hour period. In patients who have had previous anti-microbial therapy, 4-6 blood cultures may be required. The volume of blood collected is also important — in adults 5-15ml are suggested, in children 3-5ml volumes may suffice. The dilution is 1ml of blood in 10ml of broth.

Table XI

EXAMPLES OF SPECIMENS WHICH MAY BE SENT TO THE LABORATORY
TO AID IN THE DIAGNOSIS OF INFECTIOUS DISEASES

SPECIMEN	COMMENT
SPUTUM	This may be sent from patients suffering from pneumonia, from bronchopneumonia or bronchitis.
URINE	This may be sent from patients suspected of having a urinary tract infection — cystitis, pyelitis or pyelonephritis.
SWABS	These may be urethral swabs in patients with urethritis, throat swabs in patients with sore throats, wound swabs in post operative cases or pus swabs from any lesion exuding pus.
ASPIRATES	Abscesses, pleural fluid, peritoneal fluid, synovial fluid may all be submitted.
BLOOD	Blood may be submitted in order to attempt to isolate an organism or in an attempt to make a serological diagnosis.
FAECES	This may be submitted from a patient with dysentery or diarrhoea.
CEREBROSPINAL FLUID	A patient with a stiff neck and a temperature — any individual suspected of meningitis, meningo-encephalitis or even encephalitis usually is subject to a lumbar puncture.
CATHETER TIPS	The tip of any tubing which has been introduced into the patient may be submitted for culture of organisms on removal from the patient.

THE SUSPECTED ORGANISM

It is important to have a knowledge of disease and the agents causing that disease. The handling and transport of a viral specimen, a strictly anaerobic bacterial specimen and a facultative bacterial specimen are all different.

Obligate anaerobes are very susceptible to oxygen and are rapidly killed. Collection of these specimens should thus be under anaerobic conditions. The sealing of a plastic syringe with a sterile rubber stopper is only of value for a limited period as oxygen is capable of perfusing through the plastic. The specimen should thus once again be transported to the laboratory as soon as possible — a 2 hour delay may result in a valueless specimen. Certain strict anaerobes may require inocculation into prereduced media at the bedside. Viruses should be inoculated into transport media and kept at a temperature of 4°C. Amoebic dysentry is best diagnosed at the bedside by microscopy on a warm stool; in bacillary dysentry no such haste is necessary. In the diagnosis of urinary tract infection the bacterial count is critical — if the urine specimen is left at room temperature the bacteria present multiply and the number of bacteria determined by the laboratory is meaningless. Urine specimens should thus be kept in the refrigerator if a delay of greater than one hour is anticipated between collection and processing.

HANDLING OF SPECIMENS BY THE LABORATORY

A specimen is taken from a patient suspected of suffering from an infection in the hopes that the specimen will assist in the diagnosis of the disease. The specimen which is sent to the laboratory is thus one in which the clinician expects to find the organism causing the patient's illness. The handling of these specimens by the laboratory is directed towards the isolation of the pathogen. Methods of isolation are adapted to suit the suspected infectious agent. A definitive diagnosis may depend on the isolation of a pathogenic organism. If the laboratory fails to isolate the pathogen a retrospective diagnosis may often be made based on the host's specific immune response. This diagnosis depends on the host's antibody response and requires blood specimens taken early in the disease and also during convalescence. Serological diagnosis depends on the presence of a rising antibody titre.

Isolation and identification of an organism can, and often does act as a guide to treatment; diagnosis on serological grounds is at best retrospective.

THE BASIC PLAN FOR THE ISOLATION OF AN ORGANISM

(A) Direct examination

The specimen is examined directly using a microscope. The magnification required depends on the size of the organism to be studied, e.g. an electron microscope is necessary to visualise a virus. A light microscope can be used to visualise larger organisms such as bacteria or the ova produced by worms. The type of staining procedure used is determined by the physical characteristics of the organism coupled with the technique employed to visualise the pathogen.

(B) Propagation of the organism

An attempt is made to grow the organism. Different organisms have different growth requirements — some are grown on artificial chemical culture media, others require living cells. The sort of living cell required varies from tissue culture or yolk sac to the nine banded armadillo. Culture media prepared in the laboratory contains various basic substrates to which supplements or inhibitors may be added.

Culture methods are aimed at

(1) providing an environment conducive to the multiplication of the organisms present; and

(2) aiding the selection of suspicious organisms which can then be further identified.

(C) Identification

Groups of the same organism resulting from the propagation or multiplication of the organism isolated can be identified. Bacterial identification depends on the organism's metabolism, its physical and immunological constitution and, in certain cases, its ability to produce toxins. Viral identification is determined by the effect the virus has on tissue culture or other living cells, on its antigenic structure and its ability to produce classical lesions in certain laboratory animals.

(D) Quantitative testing

This is utilized when it is important to estimate the number of organisms present in a specimen. This is of no value in, for example, throat swabs; it is, however, of immense value in

(a) urine cultures where the number of organisms is used to determine whether the organism isolated is likely to be a pathogen or a contaminent;

(b) water sanitation as a public health measure.

The drinking water supplied to a population is not sterile; it contains a number of bacteria, the number of bacteria permitted must conform to certain standards as laid down by the Health Authorities.

Table XII

ORGANISMS WHICH MAY BE DEMONSTRATED IN CLINICAL SPECIMENS

	PATHOGENS	COMMENSALS
FAECES	*Vibrio cholerae*	*Escherichia coli*
	Salmonella typhi	*Streptococcus faecalis*
	Salmonella species	Clostridia
	Shigella	*Entamoeba coli*
	Entamoeba histolytica	
	Worm ova	
	Infectious hepatitis virus	
	Enteropathogenic *E. coli*	
THROAT SWABS	*Streptococcus pyogenes*	*Streptococcus viridans*
	Corynebacterium diphtheriae	Propionibacterium/
	Staphylococcus aureus	Diphtheroids
	Borrelia vincenti	*Staphylococcus epidermidis*
	Neisseria	Bacteroides
	Streptococcus pueumoniae	
	Viruses — measles	
	rubella	
	polio	
	adeno	
	parainfluenza, etc.	
URINE	*Escherichia coli*	
	Streptococcus faecalis	
	Proteus	
	Klebsiella	
	Staphylococcus	
	Pseudomonas	

	PATHOGENS	COMMENSALS
	Enterobacter	
	Salmonella typhi	
	Mycobacterium tuberculosis	
CEREBROSPINAL	*Neisseria meningitidis*	
FLUID	*Haemophilus influenzae*	
	Streptococcus pneumoniae	
	Mycobacterium tuberculosis	
	Cryptococcus neoformans	
	Listeria monocytogenes	
	Enterobacteria	
	Pseudomonas	
BLOOD	*Salmonella typhi*	
	Brucella	
	Neisseria — both *N. meningitidis* and *N. gonorrhoeae*	
	Streptococci e.g. *Strep. viridans, Strep. faecalis* and *Strep.*	
	pneumoniae	
	Hepatitis viruses — serum and infections	
	Ebstein — Barr virus (Herpes virus causing infectious mono-nucleosis)	
	Rickettsia	
	Plasmodia	
VESICLE FLUID	Variola	
	Vaccinia	
	Herpes I (oral herpes)	
	II (genital herpes)	
	III (varicella zoster)	
PUS	Staphylococcus	
	Streptococcus	
	Mycobacteria	
	Gram negative bacilli	
	Actinomycetes	
	Fungi	
SPUTUM	*Streptococcus pneumoniae*	
	Haemophilus influenzae	
	Klebsiella	
	Yersinia pestis	
	Mycobacterium tuberculosis	
	Viruses eg. adeno	

HANDLING OF A SPECIMEN FROM A PATIENT SUSPECTED OF PARASITIC INFESTATION

The type of specimen usually submitted for parasitological examination—

Stool
Urine
Blood

Stool specimens

These are first subject to direct examination.

Parasites which may be found include protozoa, e.g. amoebae, worms, cysts or ova. Examination of the stool may show the presence of adult worms or worm segments (proglottids). In tape worm infestation, proglottids may be found in the stool; in hookworm infestations, larvae may be found in the stool. The larvae and ova require magnification before they are large enough to be visualized by the human eye. Protozoa are also visualized using light microscopy.

The stool may be prepared for microscopy in two ways

(a) A direct smear may be made — a small portion of the stool is mixed in a drop of saline or iodine on a glass slide.

(b) A concentrated preparation — the parasitic ova are separated from the faecal matter using ether and centrifugation. Organisms and ova may be killed in formalin. Eosin can be added as a stain for ova.

Examination

The slide can be scanned using a magnification of 40x; final identification can be achieved at a magnification of 400x.

In the case of amoebiasis, examination of a warm stool will facilitate rapid identification of pathogenic amoebae. The amoebae responsible for amoebic dysentry display directional motility and move with 'explosive' pseudopodia; amoebae commensal in the intestine have but sluggish motility. Smears are then fixed, stained and examined to morphologically confirm the finding on the warm stool.

The identification of the parasite thus depends on the morphological characteristic of the adult parasite or the ovum.

The material to which the nurse collecting the faecal specimen is exposed, is, in most cases, infective should she ingest ova. Provided the nurse handles the faeces with reasonable care and washes adequately after collecting the specimen she is not in danger of acquiring the disease. There is, however, one exception to this rule — *Strongyloides stercoralis* ova may hatch into infective larvae in the patient's intestine or stool. These larvae are capable of penetrating intact skin and infecting the nurse who spills faeces over her hand.

Urine specimen

The ova of *Schistosoma haemotabium* may classically be found in urine. Urine may be examined directly or after centrifugation. Haematuria is commonly associated with schistomiasis.

These ova are incapable of infecting man; they require a stage of development in the snail before the organism becomes infective. Nurses are not in danger of acquiring bilharzia from their patients' excreta.

Blood specimen

Thick and thin blood smears are made and stained with one of a selected group of stains, the Romanovsky stains. The slides are examined under light microscopy. Microfilaria will be seen at a magnification of 40x, trypanosomes at 400x and plasmodia (the malaria parasite) at 1 000x.

THE HANDLING OF A SPECIMEN FOR FUNGAL EXAMINATION

The type of specimen which may be submitted for fungal examination falls into three categories —

Skin scrapings, hair or nails, i.e. skin and its appendages
Body secretions, excretions and fluids
Biopsy material.

These specimens are examined directly under light microscopy using various stains, e.g. Gram stain, Indian ink, etc. The stain selected depends on the specimen submitted and the fungus suspected. Fungi may be provisionally identified on their physical characterists and the tissue response evoked by them, e.g. sporotrichosis is identified by the presence of asteroid bodies in tissue sections. The asteroid body is a yeast form of the organism surrounded by a typical host reaction. Fungi are grown on different culture media at 37°C and 25°C. Certain fungi assume different morphological forms at body and room temperature — dimorphic fungi appear as rounded yeast forms at 37°C and as filamentous hyphae at 25°C. Fungi may be further identified by the type of spores they produce.

In the case of certain systemic fungal diseases the host's antibody response may be employed in the diagnosis of the disease. Serological diagnosis is routinely employed, e.g. in candidosis and aspergillosis.

In general, fungal specimens are not a danger to the nurse collecting the specimen as most fungi are found in the environment and only cause disease in patients with a compromised immune response. There are exceptions to this rule.

THE HANDLING OF SPECIMENS FOR BACTERIAL INVESTIGATIONS

Any fluid aspirate, secretion, excretion or catheter tip, whether used to drain urine, pus or bile, may be submitted to the laboratory for isolation of suspected bacteria.

DIRECT EXAMINATION

Two stains form the basis of direct examination. The first and most important is the Gram stain. This stain is used to divide the large majority of medically important bacteria into two groups on the basis of the organism's ability to retain a stain in the presence of decolourization by alcohol or acetone.

The Gram stain

Method:

Place a thin film of the specimen on a clean glass slide.
Fix the smear by passing the slide through the flame of a Bunsen burner.
Flood the slide with a bluish dye — crystal violet. Allow this dye to remain in contact with the smear for a few minutes.
Wash with water.

Flood the slide with Grams iodine — this mordant will penetrate the bacteria and combine with the blue-violet dye already present in the bacteria.

Wash the slide.
Decolourize using either acetone or alcohol. The exposure time is critical.

All bacteria will lose their dye if exposed to acetone of alcohol for too long a period. The optimum exposure time leads to only a certain group of bacteria consistently losing their dye. This result is reproducible. The smear is now counter-stained using a red dye — methyl red or dilute aqueous carbol fuschin.

Wash off the stain with water. Air dry. The smear is examined under oil immersion (magnification 1 000x).

Organisms which have retained initial dye stain blue and are termed Gram-positive. Those failing to retain the initial dye are stained by the counter-stain and appear red — these are termed Gram-negative.

The basic mechanism determining whether a bacterium will stain red or blue is unknown. It is postulated to be related to the structure of the cell wall.

The Gram stain in conjunction with the shape of the bacterium forms a pillar in bacteriological diagnosis.

Table XIII
BACTERIA CLASSIFIED ON THE BASIS OF THEIR MORPHOLOGY AND THE GRAM STAIN

GENERA OF GRAM-POSITIVE BACTERIA

Cocci	Streptococcus	Peptostreptococci
	Staphylococcus	Peptococci
Bacilli	Corynebacterium	
	Bacillus	
	Listeria	Clostridium

GENERA OF GRAM-NEGATIVE BACTERIA

Cocci	Neisseria	Veillonella
Bacilli	The Enterobacteriaceae —	Shigella — Escherischia
		Edwardsiella
		Salmonella — Citrobacter
		Klebsiella — Enterobacter — Serratia
		Proteus — Providentia
	Vibrio	
	Pseudomonas	
	The Parvobacteria —	Brucella
		Haemophilus
		Bordetella
		Pasturella
		Yersinia Bacteroides

The second stain of value in identification of bacteria is used in the identification of bacilli. Certain bacilli will retain a red dye even after attempts to decolourize the organism using acid and alcohol. These bacilli are called acid-fast bacilli. The stain used to detect acid-fast bacilli is the Ziehl-Neelsen stain. A thin film of the specimen is smeared onto a glass slide. Carbol fuschin is poured onto the slide and is heated until steam rises. The specimen is stained by steaming carbol fuschin (red dye) for 10 minutes. After washing in water, attempts are made to remove the red stain using both acid and alcohol. A blue counter-stain — methylene blue may be used as a background stain. Only one large group of bacilli is capable of retaining this dye — these acid-fast bacilli are called mycobacteria. (Certain actinomycetes, e.g. nocardia may also be partially acid-fast.) This stain is only of value in differentiating in acid-fast bacilli.

Stains such as Alberts stain are used for cornyebacteria, methylene blue is used for yersinia. Certain organisms fail to stain or stain poorly. In such cases dark field microscopy, phase contrast microscopy and/or fluorescent microscopy may be employed.

Culture

Bacteria are grown on various artificial culture media. Media is the term used to describe the nutrient mixtures used for the cultivation of bacteria. For culture results to be meaningful a knowledge of the normal flora of the site from which the specimen has been taken is essential. Media supply a physical and chemical environment suitable for growth of bacteria. The physical environment may be liquid, semi-solid or solid. The solid media is dependent for its solidity on an agar base. Agar consists of a polysaccharide network which acts as a sponge holding water in its intersticies. The percentage composition of water present determines if the agar is solid or semi-solid. Agar is non-toxic to bacteria, it melts at 90°C and remains a liquid on cooling until the temperature drops to 45-50°C. Additives or substrates that are relatively heat labile can therefore be added at a temperature of 50°C. Agar at 37°C (i.e. at the temperature at which most laboratory incubators are set) is a solid. The chemical environment is composed of nutrients required for bacterial growth.

Basic media

This supplies the essential nutrients required for the growth of bacteria. Examples include — meat, tryptose digests, peptone water, nutrient broth.

A basic nutrient medium is one which must contain a hydrogen donor and a hydrogen acceptor amongst its constituents. Compounds which are classified as hydrogen donors or oxidizable substances are required as an energy source. Compounds capable of accepting hydrogen are required for this purpose during energy yielding oxidation — reduction reactions. In the case of aerobic organisms, gaseous oxygen acts as the hydrogen acceptor. Organic compounds or inorganic substances, e.g. sulphate, nitrate or carbonate may act as hydrogen acceptors in metabolism of anaerobic organisms. Basic nutrient media must contain a carbon and a nitrogen source. It must also supply a variety of minerals including iron, potassium and magnesium for the growth of the organism.

Any basic nutrient medium may be adapted and changed into a selective medium by the addition of substances inhibitory to certain micro-organisms. The selective media so produced is capable of inhibiting the growth of certain organisms and thus facilitating the growth of others.

Selective media

This medium is used when the clinical specimen submitted is suspected of containing a small number of pathogens and a large number of commensal organisms. The suspected pathogen may be given an environmental advantage by the addition of a substance which is inhibitory to the commensal organisms but which has little influence on its own metabolism. Examples of selective media include bile salt agar, agar with a high saline content, e.g. Chapman's agar, and medium with a high pH, e.g. alkaline peptone water.

Chapman's agar is inhibitory to most bacteria due to its high salt content. Staphylococci can grow in the presence of this saline content and Chapman's agar is thus a selective medium for staphylococci.

Alkaline peptone water permits the multiplication of *Vibrio cholerae* but inhibits most other intestinal bacteria.

Enriched media

This media is supplemented with selected substances. It is used to encourage the growth of bacteria genetically unable to synthesise certain building blocks. For example — blood agar, haemolysed blood agar.

Indicator media

The incorporation of certain substrates into the medium can lead to the detection of the presence of various enzymes in the bacteria grown. Haemolysin is detected on blood agar; the metabolism of lactose to lactic acid is detected by a change in the colour of a pH sensitive dye.

The ability of certain members of the intestinal flora to ferment lactose is detected by a colour change from yellowish to pink. These organisms can therefore be excluded as possible pathogens in adult diarrhoea at a relatively early stage of specimen analysis.

The pH, moisture, type of nutrients, and the presence or absence of oxygen are all factors which modify the growth of organisms.

An adequate supply of oxygen to obligate aerobes can present a problem. In fact the factor limiting growth may be the oxygen content of the medium. In liquid media oxygen may be supplied by mixing a stream of oxygen into the culture. Obligate anaerobes have the opposite problem. Here oxygen must be removed from the medium. In liquid media a strong reducing agent, e.g. sodium thioglycollate may be added. Media may be placed in sealed containers which have been depleted of oxygen. These containers may have their oxygen removed by evacuation of the container or by means of a chemical reaction which consumes the free oxygen.

The result of culturing a specimen can vary

(1) A specimen may contain a single bacterium — this is the usual result when the specimen is taken from a normally sterile site. Provided that the specimen has not been contaminated the organism isolated can be assumed to be the pathogen responsible for the patient's disease.

(2) A specimen may contain a number of bacteria — normal flora must be recognised and excluded from those colonies which require further investigation. A colony is a large number of bacteria which are clustered together in a group and form the progeny of a single

Figure 9
BACTERIAL CULTURE AND IDENTIFICATION OF E. coli

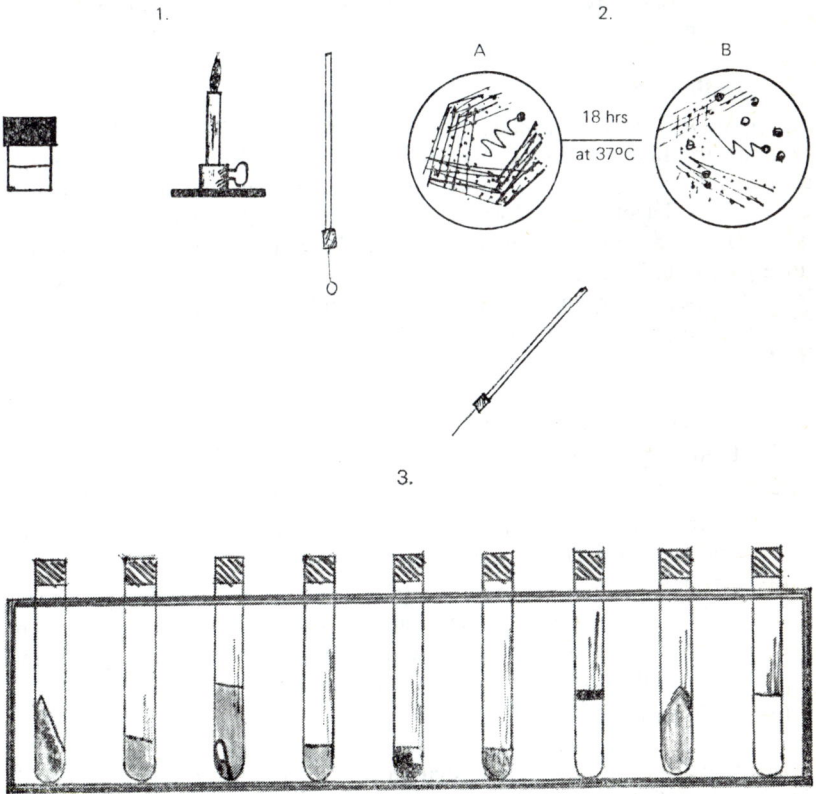

1. Flame the bacterial loop, allow it to cool and plant a loopful of specimen on agar plate 'A'.
2. Plate out for single colonies.
3. Pick a single colony off plate 'B' and plant it in biochemical test media. After overnight incubation at 37°C read the organism's biochemical profile according to the colour change induced in the media.

bacterium. In view of this it is imperative that the clinical staff facilitate the laboratory and provide an accurate note of the anatomical site from which the specimen was obtained. Knowledge of the provisional diagnosis can also facilitate laboratory work in the choice of selective media. Basic procedures are routinely carried out in the laboratory — clinical information can in certain cases alter this routine to the benefit of the patient, the doctor and the laboratory.

Culture results in a three-fold harvest

(*a*) Certain colonies suspected of being pathogenic in that anatomical site are isolated.

(*b*) A pure culture of the suspected organism has been obtained.

(*c*) Sufficient material for further identification is available. Culture provides pure material on which identification tests can be performed.

Identification

A single organism multiplies to form a colony — identification of the original organism isolated can now be achieved by subjecting its progeny to a variety of tests. The organism is grown in a specific system which is adapted to detect a secretory product or metabolite produced by that organism. The ability of an organism to ferment certain sugars, to produce gas, to utilize certain substrates and to excrete various by-products leads to specific organisms producing specific biochemical profiles. The biochemical pattern so produced is a corner stone in the identification of bacteria.

Organisms may thus be identified by —

(1) their morphology, staining characteristics and motility;

(2) their capacity for aerobic, anaerobic or facultative growth;

(3) their ability to grow on simple media or their requirement for selective or enriched media;

(4) Biochemical pathways form a pattern characteristic of certain organisms. Organisms may be identified by their specific requirement for certain factors, by their ability to secrete certain enzymes and by the end products of their metabolic pathways;

(5) their antigenic structure.

Identification of the antigenic structure of the organism may take classification out of the stage of genus and species recognition into the realm of strain identification. Identification of an organism by means of its antigenic structure requires the use of a known antisera (antibody) which will react specifically with that organism. A specific reaction between a known and an unknown when an antigen and antibody are involved results in identification of the unknown.

If the laboratory has failed to isolate the pathogenic organism its identity may be inferred by studying the host's response to infection by that organism. A specific reaction between the host's antibody and a known organism is diagnostic of previous exposure of the host to that organism. If at the beginning of the illness the patient's blood contained no antibodies against an organism and during this patient's convalescence antibodies to that organism were detected then one can conclude that that species of organism was responsible for the patient's recent illness. The clinical picture would limit the number of suspected causative organisms. Only the range of organisms suggested by the clinical picture would be tested against the host's serum for the presence of antibody.

Drug sensitivity testing

Pure cultures of the pathogen are tested *in vitro* against various antimicrobial agents. The laboratory can thus provide a guide to the treatment of choice for various bacterial infections.

The organism isolated may be tested against a range of anti-microbial agents. The anti-microbial agents capable of inhibiting growth of the bacterium in the laboratory are selected as the agents of choice for the treatment of that bacterial infection in the patient. If the anti-microbial agent fails to inhibit the growth of the organism in the laboratory it is unlikely to be of value in inhibiting the growth of the organism in the patient. In the laboratory one of the techniques employed to assess drug sensitivity uses discs. The drugs to be tested are impregnated onto paper discs. The disc is incubated overnight on a planted culture plate. If the drug is capable of inhibiting growth a zone free of bacterial growth is found around the disc. In cases where the organisms is resistant to the drug the bacteria grow right up to the edge of the disc.

Biological tests

A variety of animals may be used to assist in the study of bacteria. The differentiation of mycobacteria according to their ability to infect a variety of laboratory animals assists in the definitive identification and differentiation of *Mycobacterium tuberculosis*. A Gram-positive bacillus providing a classical clinical picture in mice may be identified as *Clostridium tetani*. Protection of a second control mouse by tetanus antiserum confirms this result. Stimulation of the animal's immune system by injection of an unknown organism can lead to a diagnosis based on its antibody response.

Biological tests still have a limited but important role in bacteriology. They have largely been replaced by improved biochemical techniques. Biological tests are costly and unpopular with the female laboratory technicians.

LABORATORY HANDLING OF SPECIMENS SUBMITTED FOR VIRAL PATHOGENS

The isolation of viruses from clinical specimens is an expensive and complicated procedure. Viral isolation is thus reserved for specific occasions.

These occasions arise if —

(i) the virus presents a public health hazard, e.g. smallpox or lassa fever outbreaks.

(ii) The suspected virus is amenable to therapy, in other words, when a definitive diagnosis will alter the treatment and/or management of a case.

(iii) The virus is of academic interest. Viruses are isolated in order to identify new agents of disease and in order to better classify viruses already associated with disease.

DIRECT EXAMINATION

Electron microscopy is of value in the rapid confirmation of a clinical diagnosis in certain cases, e.g. confirmation of a case of smallpox. Light microscopy may also be used in the diagnosis of viral diseases. The virus itself is too small to be visualized using light microscopy, thus the light microscopic diagnosis of viral diseases depends on the tissue response of the host to the viral infection. Cytomegalovirus is suspected when large intranuclear inclusions are seen, smallpox when Guarneiri bodies, and rabies when Negri bodies are seen. Immunofluorescence using fluorescent antibody may also be of value in the diagnosis of viral disease.

Table XIV

CELLULAR CHANGES INDUCED BY VIRAL INFECTIONS

The following cellular changes are seen on light microscopy.
Viruses producing inclusion bodies in host cells:

(a) Intra-nuclear	Herpes (not Ebstein-Barr virus)	
	Yellow fever (Brain)	
	Adenovirus	
(b) Intra-cytoplasmic	Rabies	
	Poxvirus	
	Parainfluenza, types I and II	
	Respiratory syncitial virus	
(c) Intra-cytoplasmic and intra-nuclear inclusions	Influenza B	
	Parainfluenza, type III	
	Mumps	
	Measles	
	Yellow fever (liver)	

Viruses causing giant cell formation:

Herpes I, II, III
Parainfluenza, type II
Measles
Mumps
Respiratory syncitial

VIRAL PROPAGATION

Three systems have been employed for viral propagation. These are tissue culture, egg inoculation and animal, e.g. mice inoculation. As different viruses are best adapted to one of these systems, it is helpful for the laboratory to select the system to be used on the basis of the clinician's provisional diagnosis.

Specimens should reach the laboratory without delay. Transport should be at 4°C. If a delay in delivery is anticipated the specimen should be frozen at −20°C. Specimens for viral isolation should be transported in special transport media. Antibiotics are usually part of this medium. Specimens may range from tissue biopsies to vesicle fluid, to upper respiratory tract secretions. Many of these specimens are contaminated by bacteria and thus it is important to remove these contaminants prior to inoculation. Antibiotics, bacterial filters and differential centrifugation may be used to achieve a pure viral inoculum.

The choice of the propagation system depends on the suspected pathogen and hence on the clinical picture. Laboratory animals used for inoculation of viruses include guinea pigs, mice and rabbits.

Table XV

EXAMPLES OF VIRAL PROPAGATION SYSTEMS

(1) Egg inoculation	— Pox viruses	
	Influenza	
	Mumps	
	Rabies	
(2) Tissue culture	— On monkey kidney	Polio
		Echo
		Influenza A and B
		Parainfluenza, types 1-4
		Measles
		Mumps
		Respiratory syncitial
	— On human embryonic fibroblasts	Herpes, types I, II, III, V
	— On lymphocytes	Herpes IV
(3) Animal inoculation	— Baby mice	Coxsackie A and B
	— Adult mice	Arboviruses
		Arenaviruses

The site of inoculation depends on the laboratory animal chosen and the pathogen suspected. Diagnosis of disease depends on the development of disease in that animal or the production of a rising antibody titre by that animal. All animals are subject to autopsies and histological diagnosis may be of further value.

Cell cultures when inoculated with a viral suspension undergo a variety of changes depending on the type of virus inoculated, e.g.

   (i) A cytopathic effect — the infected cells undergo characteristic degenerative changes in either the nucleus, e.g. herpes viruses; the cytoplasm, e.g. respiratory syncitial virus, or both, e.g. the mumps virus.

  (ii) Syncitial formation — the formation of multinucleate giant cells is characteristic, e.g. of measles.

 (iii) Interference — certain viruses produce no histologically detectable changes but can prevent superinfection of the tissue culture cells by a second known virus which does produce cytopathic changes. Rubella produces no histological changes but decreases the rate of growth and multiplication of infected cells.

(iv) Haemadsorption — influenza virus alters the surface of tissue culture cells so that red blood cells become adsorbed onto the surface of the tissue culture cells.

Embyronated eggs are inoculated into certain selected sites, e.g. the chorioallantoic membrane is inoculated if smallpox is suspected, the amniotic sac is inoculated if influenza is suspected.

The pattern of infection, the changes induced in these systems and the ability of certain viruses to infect one system only, leads to a characteristic pattern being associated with any virus.

Therapy for viral disease is limited, isolation techniques are difficult and costly. Retrospective diagnosis has thus assumed an important rôle in viral diseases. Here the specific host response as detected by antibody production in response to the viral infection is diagnostic. Two blood samples — an acute plus a convalescent sample are tested for the unknown antibody against known virus. Interaction between the unknown antibody and the known antigen (virus) leads to identification of the unknown. The clinician can then deduce to which virus the patient has been exposed. A rising antibody titre, i.e. an increase in the specific host response to that particular virus, is diagnostic of previous recent acute infection by that virus.

Table XVI
HINTS ON SPECIMEN COLLECTION FOR NURSES

1. A specimen for microbacteriological examination is potentially dangerous.
2. Where possible collect the specimen directly into the container supplied by the laboratory.
3. Take care not to contaminate specimens during or after collection.
4. No specimens for bacteriology should be collected in formalin, alcohol or any other disinfectant.
5. All specimens must reach the laboratory with *minimal* delay. The value of the microbiological report decreases as the time period between specimen collection and laboratory processing increases.

Specimens frequently collected by the nursing staff:

Urine — Mid-stream clean voided specimen.
Early morning urine.
Refrigerated if a delay of more than 1 hour is anticipated between collection of specimen and arrival at the laboratory.

Sputum — Deep cough specimen.
Early morning.

Faeces — Select suspicious areas, e.g. blood stains, mucus, for submission to the laboratory.

Swabs — A dry swab of a dry lesion is of little value.
A swab which takes longer than one hour to reach the laboratory is of limited value.

SUMMARY

AIM

To find (isolate), recognise (identify) and often to grow (culture) the agent causing the patient's disease.

METHOD

(a) Collection of specimens —
    the correct specimen
    an adequately labelled specimen
    rapid transport to the laboratory

(b) Laboratory methods —
    direct examination, magnification required
    wet or dry preparation
    staining — dye, immunofluorescence

Value

To attempt to visualize an aetiological agent and/or the host's response at a cellular level. Adequate visualization may be diagnostic. N.B. parasitic diseases.

(c) Propagation of the organism —
    artificial media with nutritional supplementation
    living cells

Value

In identifying the optimal system and conditions for propagation or multiplication of the organism —
    material for future tests becomes available
    early identification is begun
    proof that a viable agent is present is obtained
    the separation of commensal and pathogen is begun

(d) Further identification —
    biochemical tests
    serological tests

Value

Accurate identification can be of importance —

(a) as a public health measure in tracing of outbreaks;
(b) in the initial diagnosis of disease in an individual;
(c) in differentiating between relapses and reinfections in the patient; and
(d) from an academic point of view.

The request for MCS

When sent to a bacteriology department, this leads to the following responses:

M = microscopy   A direct examination of the specimen will show if bacteria are present. These may be further identified as cocci or bacilli, as Gram-positive, Gram-negative or as acid-fast.

C = culture   This involves growth of all the organisms present and the selection of organisms suspected of being pathogens for further identification.

S = sensitivity   This is a reflection of the spectrum of antimicrobial agents to which the pathogen is sensitive.

Table XVII
THE LABORATORY EXAMINATION OF SPECIMENS

A. PARASITES

Blood specimens —
    Thick smears
    Thin smears
    Selective staining
Urine —
    Direct
    Concentrated specimen
Faeces —
    Direct — Wet preparation
        Dry preparation
    Stain — Iodine
        Eosin

Organisms suspected —
    Plasmodia
    Microfilaria
    Trypanosomes
Look for —
    Ova

Look for —
    Ova and Larvae — Microscopic
    Worm — Macroscopic

B. FUNGI

I   Direct Examination   — Light microscopic examination of skin scraping
                                   Tissues sections
                                   Secretions

II   Culture — antibiotics may be incorporated into the media

III   Identification   — Cultural morphology at 25°C
                                       and 37°C
                                 Biochemical tests
                                 Serological tests

C. BACTERIA

I   Direct Examination   —(a)   Stain — Gram stain
                                           Ziehl-Neelsen
                                         Other
                       (b)   Light Microscopy
                                         Fluorescent Microscopy
                                       Dark Field Microscopy

II   Culture   — Media — Solid
                               Liquid
    (a)   Basic Media — most organisms grow on this
    (b)   Selective Media — inhibitory substances prevent overgrowth by certain organisms
    (c)   Enriched Media — additives stimulate the growth of certain organisms
    (d)   Indicator Media — an aid to early preliminary grouping of organisms

III   Identification —
    (a)   Cultural Morphology
    (b)   Growth characteristics on various media
    (c)   Biochemical tests designed to identify the metabolic pattern of an organism
    (d)   Serotype — identify surface antigenic structure of the organism
    (e)   Phage type — identify the organism's susceptibility to known phages
    (f)   Colicine/Pyocine typing — identify susceptibility to bacterio-toxic substances secreted by particular organisms.

(*a*) to (*c*) = usually leads to the identity of genus and species.
After identification of genus and species proceed selectively to (*d*), (*e*) or (*f*) for strain identification.

IV Sensitivity testing —
The pathogenic organism isolated in II is tested for susceptibility to a range of anti-microbial agents.
If growth of the organism is inhibited, this anti-microbial agent may be used in the treatment of the patient from whom this specimen was obtained.
If growth of the organism is unimpaired, this drug should not be used to treat the patient.

V Biological —
Laboratory animals used — Guinea pigs
                                 Mice
                                 Rabbits

Used (*a*) In the identification and isolation of the organism
       e.g. *Mycobacterium tuberculosis*
           Yersinia pestis

   (*b*) In the identification of toxin production
       e.g. *Clostridium tetani*
           Corynebacterium diphtheriae

   (*c*) In the identification of an unknown organism by antibody production
       e.g. *Brucella abortus*
           Brucella melitensis

D. VIRUSES

I Direct Examination   — Light Microscopy — cellular changes
                                 Electron Microscopy — visualization of the virus

II Propagation   — Cell free media of no value
                                 Animals or tissue culture

III Identification   — Histological changes
                                 Serological studies

MAGNIFICATION

Magnification is an apparent increase in the size of an object. This increase in size is achieved by the use of light or electron beams in conjunction with a system of lenses. The size increase is purely a visual phenomenon. It is difficult to really comprehend magnification:

Table XVIII

MAGNIFICATION IN PERSPECTIVE

	ACTUAL SIZE	LIGHT x 1 000	MICROSCOPY ELECTRON x 50 000	x 500 000
Man — height	1,8m	1,8Km	90Km	900Km
Erythrocyte	8μm	8mm	40cm	4m
Fungus				
e.g. yeast	10μm	1cm	50cm	5m
Bacterium				
e.g. coccus	1μm	1mm	5cm	50cm
Virus—small	20nm	20μm	1mm	1cm
large	300nm	0,3mm	1,5cm	15cm

CHAPTER 4

Parasites, Bacteria and Viruses

THE WORMS

PLATYHELMINTHS

Flat worms which may affect man's health are the trematodes or 'flukes' and the cestodes or 'tape-worms'.

THE TREMATODES

There are two groups of trematodes —

(*a*) Those which are hermaphrodites (i.e. male and female sex organs are present in the same worm)

     e.g. *Paragonimus westermanni* — the lung fluke
         Clonorchis senensis   — the Chinese liver fluke
         Fasciola hepatica   — the liver fluke

Figure 10
A GENERAL LIFE-CYCLE FOR TREMATODES

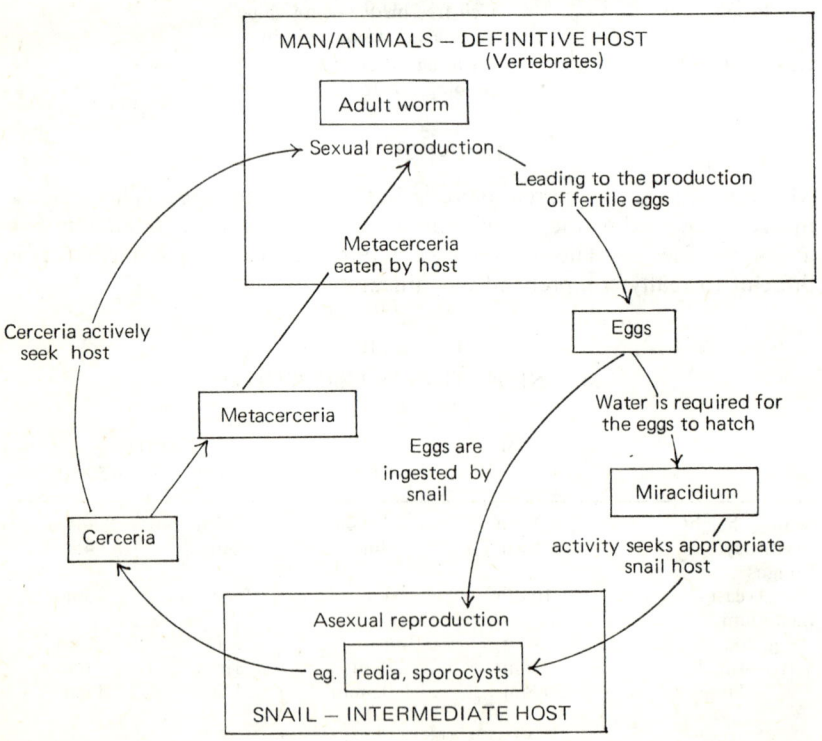

(b) Those which are non-hermaphrodite (i.e. worms which are either male or female) — e.g. Schistosomes — the blood fluke.

Distinguishing features in the trematode life cycle include the following:
(i) They have both vertebrate and invertebrate hosts participating in their life cycle.
(ii) They have a free living stage in their life cycle.
(iii) They reproduce both sexually and asexually at different stages of their life cycle. The host in which sexual reproduction of a parasite occurs is the definitive host; asexual reproduction occurs in the intermediate host.
(iv) In the case of *Clonorchis senensis* the eggs are ingested by the snail, in the case of all the other trematodes mentioned the miracidia actively penetrate the snail's foot or head.
(v) The cerceria of the schistosomes actively penetrate the vertebrate host; other cerceria encyst as metacerceria and are ingested by the definitive vertebrate host.
(vi) The trematodes are selective in their choice of hosts.

Table XIX

MORE IMPORTANT FEATURES OF MEDICALLY IMPORTANT TREMATODES

ORGANISM	ADULT WORM	SNAIL SPECIES	METACERCERIA ENCYST ON	TARGET ORGAN
NON-HERMAPHRODITE				
S.mansoni	man, baboon	Biomphalaria	—	bowel
S.haematobium	man	Bulinus	—	bladder
S.japonicum	man, domestic animals	Oncomylania	—	abdominal
HERMAPHRODITE				
Clonorchis senensis	dog, cat	Parafossarula	gills of fish	biliary system
Opisthorcis phelenus	cat	Bithynia	muscles of fish	biliary system
Paragonimus westermanni	rats, carnivors	Melania	fresh water crabs	lung
Fasciola hepatica	sheep, herbivors	Lymnaeae	grass	liver

Pathology

Disease can be due to:
(i) The presence of the worm — the worm may cause obstruction, e.g. of the bile duct. The adult worm during its migration through the body of the host may get lost and cause local lesions in the brain.
(ii) The eggs — the immune response of the host is more marked towards the eggs than towards the adult worm. Death of the eggs releases antigen and the host responds with granuloma formation. Fibrosis can result in stricture formation and loss of functional parenchymatous tissue.

Diagnosis

A definitive diagnosis is possible if ova are observed in urine, faeces or sputum. Each trematode produces a characteristic ovum. As eggs are produced by mature worms there is a time lapse between exposure, infection and the production of eggs, e.g. in the case of *Schistosoma mansoni* this delay is 6-8 weeks; in the case of *Schistosoma haematobium* this delay is 13 weeks. Complement fixation tests are also used.

Control and prevention

These worms have a complex life cycle. They require the presence of —

    (i) a vertebrate host;

    (ii) an invertebrate snail host;

    (iii) the correct environment — water for the eggs to hatch, grass on which the metacerceria may encyst, etc.

    Approach to prevention may be as follows:

    (i) Treatment of the disease in the vertebrate host and prevent reinfection of this host.

    (ii) Kill snail hosts and break the life cycle required for the propagation of these parasites.

    (iii) Separate the vertebrate host and his excreta from snails. Each of these approaches enjoys a measure of success.

Bilharzia

Bilharzia or schistosomiasis is an important disease in Southern Africa. Infection by both *Schistosoma haematobium* and *Schistosoma mansoni* may occur simultaneously in the same individual. *Schistosoma haematobium* is found throughout Africa, the distribution of *Schistosoma mansoni* is more patchy.

The presence of bilharzia in an area depends on the presence of snails and water. Snails die in rivers in which the temperature is between 0-5°C for five days. Snails are therefore not found in rivers above 4 000 feet. In South Africa bathing is safe in rivers that flow west into the Atlantic Ocean and in those rivers flowing into the Indian Ocean between Cape Point and Plettenberg Bay.

Figure 11
THE CESTODES

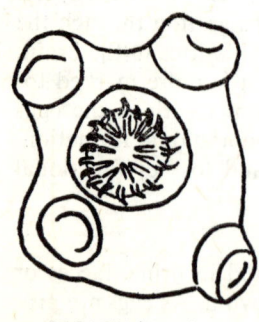

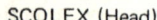

SCOLEX (Head)   ADULT WORM SHOWING PROGLOTTIDS

THE CESTODES

The cestodes or tape worms have a body consisting of segments or proglottids. Each proglottid develops from a growth zone near the 'head' or scolex of the worm. As the proglottid matures it passes through a male and then a female phase. By the time the proglottid has been displaced to the distal end of the worm it consists of a "bag of eggs". The proglottid is distended by eggs contained in its uterine branches. This mature proglottid is expelled in the faeces of the host or it may crawl out of the host's anus.

Cestodes have no free living stage. The adult worm lives in the small intestine of the definitive host. The larval stage migrates and forms cysts in the muscle or parenchymal tissue of the intermediate host.

Figure 12
THE CESTODE LIFE CYCLE

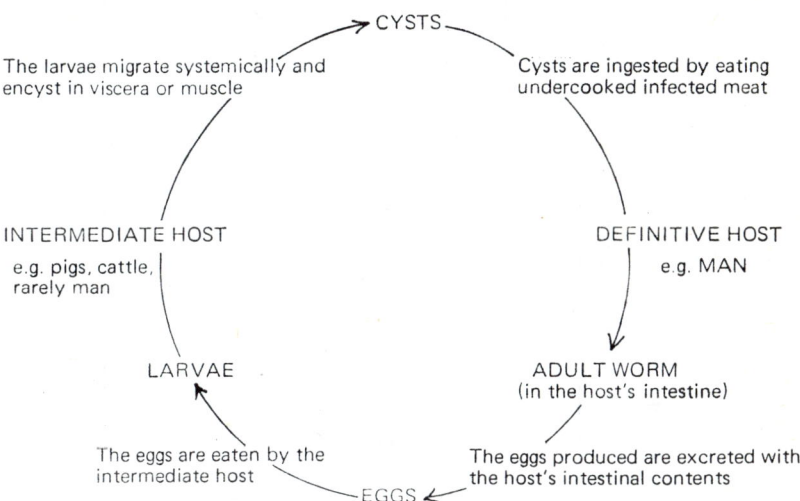

Basic Life Cycle:

CYSTS

The larvae migrate systemically and encyst in viscera or muscle

Cysts are ingested by eating undercooked infected meat

INTERMEDIATE HOST
e.g. pigs, cattle, rarely man

DEFINITIVE HOST
e.g. MAN

LARVAE

ADULT WORM
(in the host's intestine)

The eggs are eaten by the intermediate host

The eggs produced are excreted with the host's intestinal contents

EGGS

Pathology

The disease can be due to —

(a) The presence of the worm — the adult worm is found in the intestine of the host. Its eggs are not trapped in the host's tissues but are freely excreted along with the faecal mass. Side effects caused by the worm can occur as a result of competition for nutrients, e.g. vitamin B_{12}. Absorption of metabolites provided by the worm can lead to psychological effects in the host. The observation of a proglottid in the host's stool may also lead to psychological symptons. Certain 'workers' attempted to introduce larval tapeworm tablets as a novel means of slimming. This slimming technique came to an inglorious end when tablets left lying in the sunlight started to move.

Table XX

LISTING THE MORE IMPORTANT FEATURES OF MEDICALLY IMPORTANT CESTODES

ORGANISM	DEFINITIVE HOST	INTERMEDIATE HOST	CYST	DISEASE IN MAN
Taenia solium	man	pig, occasionally man	cysticercus	Cysticercosis
Taenia saginata	man	cattle	cysticercus	—
Taenia multiceps	dog, cat	herbivorous animal, occasionally man	coenurus	Coenurus cerebralis
Echinococcus granulosus	canines, e.g. jackal	herbivorous animal, occasionally man	hydatid	Hydatid disease

In the above cases when the adult worm is found in man it is well tolerated.

WORM INFESTATIONS PREDOMINATING IN CHILDREN				DISEASE DUE TO ADULT WORM
Dibothriocephalus latus	carnivor e.g. jackal, man	fish	pleurocercoid	anaemia (B_{12} deficiency) CYSTS $\rightarrow$ SPARGANOSIS
Dipyllidium canicum	dog	dog flea	cysticercoid	psychological effects
Hymenolepis nana	birds, rodents	nil or insects	cysticercoid	malaise, occasionally diarrhoea

(b) The presence of the larval cyst — the cysts can lead to serious complications. If man ingests cestode eggs, the eggs can hatch in his intestine. The larvae migrate to various viscera and cysts are formed. These cysts, depending on their anatomical site, can cause various effects. If a cyst is present in the brain it may block drainage of the cerebro-spinal fluid causing raised intracranial pressure; it may on death of the larvae calcify and cause epilepsy. Removal of the cysts from brain, liver, etc., is a dangerous procedure as rupture of a viable cyst releases one or more larvae capable of developing into egg producing adults in the central nervous system or abdominal cavity.

Diagnosis

In general tapeworm ova can be differentiated from other ova by the presence of hooklets. Identification of the type of cestode by examination of the ovum is only possible in certain cases.

Other methods of diagnosing cestodes includes examination of any proglottids passed in the faeces. Cysts squashed between two glass slides can be identified by the number and type of scolices present.

Prevention and control

Treatment of *Taenia saginata* or *Taenia solium* in man results in death of the adult worm. The worm releases its hold on the intestine and is passed out of the intestine by peristalsis. *Taenia solium* may respond to certain therapy by releasing its ova into the lumen of the intestine. Those eggs which are transported by retrograde peristalsis to the stomach hatch in the host's intestine, and release their larvae. Migration of these larvae causes cysticercosis. In cases of cestode infestation a constipated bowel should be evacuated prior to treatment.

Prevention of disease is by adequate control and condemnation of infected meat. Treatment of the cyst, other than surgical excision, is contra-indicated as the host's immune response to the dead larva is exaggerated. Treatment of a cerebral cyst can precipitate epilepsy.

Certain of the cestodes are acquired by children during their contact with infected pets.

THE NEMATODES

The nematodes are also called "round worms". Between the egg and adult stages their life cycle involves a number of different larval stages. Transmission varies:

(a) Certain eggs are transmitted directly from one host to the next by the faecal-oral route, e.g. the pinworm.

(b) Other eggs require a stage of maturation in soil. They hatch to form larvae which actively penetrate the skin of the new host, e.g. hookworms.

(c) Certain nematodes, the filaria, are transmitted by arthropods, e.g. *Loa loa*.

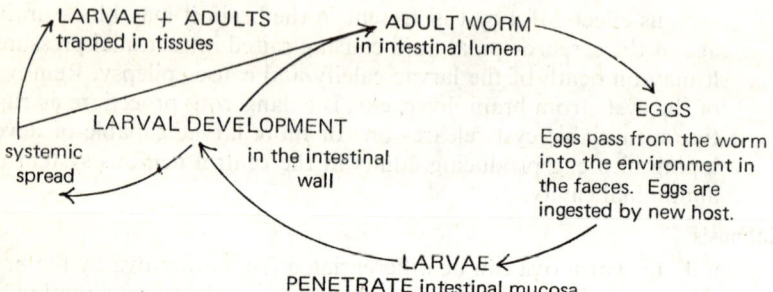

Figure 13
THE LIFE CYCLE OF NEMATODES SPREAD BY THE FAECAL-ORAL ROUTE

Nematodes transmitted by the faecal-oral route

Trichuris trichura: The Whip worm

Enterobius vermicularis: The Pinworm

Both these round worms are confined to the intestine. The adults are frequently found in the caecum. The female pinworm migrates out of the anus and deposits her eggs in the peri-anal region — this results in pruritis ani. Children are frequently infested by this worm. When one member of a family becomes infested it is necessary to treat the whole family — including father. The eggs shed from the child's anal area are small light-weight eggs which float and land on many objects in the environment.

Trichuris infestation is usually asymptomatic — only heavy infestations are accompanied by symptoms. Man is the definitive host in the case of both trichuris and enterobius.

The definitive host for *Ascaris lumbricoides* is man; for *Toxocara canis*, the dog and for *Toxocara cati*, the cat. The larvae of these worms undergo a systemic migration prior to settling in the intestinal lumen of their natural host. When man ingests the eggs of toxocara the larvae fail to migrate back to the intestine and become lodged in the visera. *Toxocara canis* and *Toxocara cati*, the dog and cat ascarids, cause viseral larva migrans in man.

Nematodes requiring ingestion of eggs or larvae in animal tissue for transmission

Capillaria hepatica and *Trichinella spiralis* are transmitted by the consumption of infected animal tissue.

Inadequately cooked pork is a vehicle for the transmission of *Trichinella spiralis*. The larvae are released from their cysts on exposure to the digestive juices of the host's intestine. The adults mate in the upper gastrointestinal tract and produce larvae which penetrate the intestine and migrate to the host's skeletal muscle. Cold storage at −18°C for at least two weeks is required to kill the larvae in pork.

Both *Trichinella spiralis* and *Capillaria hepatica* are not natural parasites of man. They are classified amongst the zoonoses.

Capillaria hepatica is a nematode of rodents. Children are occasionally infected. Infection results from the ingestion of eggs found in rat faeces. These eggs hatch, the larvae migrate to the liver and the adults lay their eggs in the liver. The infected child will thus never excrete the ova of this worm in the faeces. If the child ingests eggs found in rat liver, not faeces, then the ingested eggs will be excreted in that child's faeces. In this case the child is the paratenic host or the carrier. These eggs are non-invasive as the egg requires exposure to digestive enzymes plus a time lapse before the larvae can be released. The carrier therefore excretes eggs in his faeces. Only after the eggs have been passed through the gastro-intestinal tract are they infective on subsequent ingestion.

Figure 14
A TYPICAL LIFE CYCLE OF NEMATODES
CAPABLE OF PERCUTANEOUS INVASION

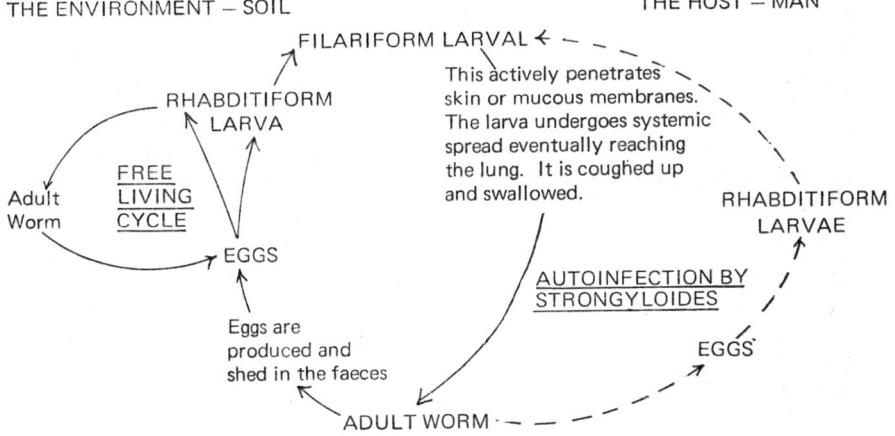

Nematodes transmitted by active percutaneous larval penetration
Strongyloides stercoralis, *Ancylostoma duodenale* and *Necator americanus* all fall into this group.

Hookworms are recognised as an important cause of anaemia in the tropics. They require a maturation phase in soil during which they undergo a free living larval stage. The definitive host is man.

Strongyloides may cut short its life cycle. Instead of the larvae developing in the soil they may become invasive while still in the host's intestine. Strongyloides can thus auto-infect the host — as strongyloides is capable of multiplication within the same host, suppression of the host immune response is dangerous. Immunosuppression can permit excessive multiplication of this worm in the host. Of all the worms already mentioned, strongyloides is the only one capable of multiplying within the host — this means that infection by strongyloides has graver implications from the point of view of worm load.

Ancylostoma braziliensis, the dog hookworm, causes sandworm in man. The larva attempts to penetrate the skin of the wrong host but finds itself incapable of penetrating the dermis. The larva therefore migrates through the skin leaving in its wake an allergic erythrematous streak. Sandworm is also called cutaneous larva migrans.

Nematodes injected percutaneously into vertebrate hosts

The filarial worms are mainly found in tropical and sub-tropical areas.

Wucheria bancrofti is spread by mosquitoes and causes lymphadenitis and elephantiasis in man.

Loa-loa is spread by chrysops, a fly, and this worm causes calabar swellings. Loaiasis manifests itself by migratory sub-cutaneous oedema and erythrema.

Onchocerca volvulus is spread by simulium — the black fly. The species of fly which carries oncocercus is called *Simulium damnosum*. Onchocerciasis is a disease which manifests itself as subcutaneous nodules, caused by the adults, and retinal damage culminating in blindness caused by the microfilaria. River blindness is the name given by local people to this disease.

Acanthocheilonema perstans is spread by culicoides, the biting midge. This worm has no clear association with disease but may cause eosinophilia.

Female filarial worms are either viviparous, laying embryonated eggs, or ovoviviparous discharging their larvae directly into the host's blood stream. The larvae are called microfilariae. The microfilaria, except for those of onchocercus, circulate in the blood and are picked up by a biting arthropod. The larvae develop further in the arthropod host and when mature are injected by the arthropod through the skin of a new vertebrate host. Man can act as the definitive host for all the filaria mentioned. The adult worms settle in the peritoneal cavity in the case of *Acanthocheilonema*

Figure 15
A GENERAL VIEW OF A FILARIAL LIFE CYCLE

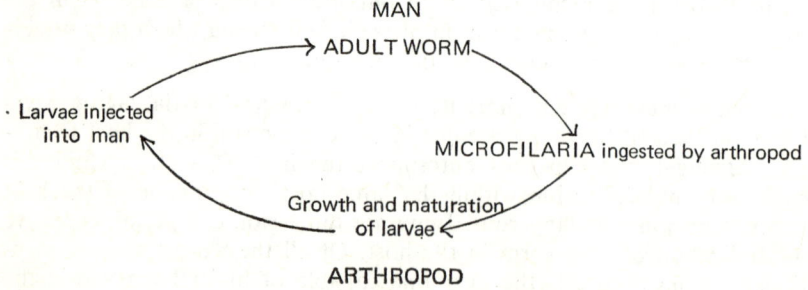

MAN

ADULT WORM

· Larvae injected into man

MICROFILARIA ingested by arthropod

Growth and maturation of larvae

ARTHROPOD

perstans, in the lymphatics or lymph nodes in the case of *Wucheria bancrofti* and are found subcutaneously in both oncercerciasis and loaiasis. The microfilaria are found in the blood, except in the case of onchocerciasis where they are found in the skin.

The host's response plays an important role in the disease caused by the filarial worms and their larvae, the microfilaria. Allergy is a major factor in the pathogenesis of river blindness, elephantiasis and calabar swellings. Eosinophilia is often associated with systemic nematode invasion.

Diagnosis of nematode worms

(i) The eggs — in many cases microscopic examination of the faeces will lead to the demonstration of ova in individuals infected with nematode worms. Many nematodes produce distinct ova, e.g. ascaris, trichuris, enterobius.

(ii) The larvae — hookworms and strongyloides cannot be distinguished from one another on the appearance of their ova — examnation of the larvae will, however, enable one to distinguish between these worms. The hookworms are distinguished by morphological differences between their larvae, while strongyloides is identified by the presence of larvae in a fresh stool.

Microfilaria can be identified according to —

(*a*) the arrangement of their nuclei; and

(*b*) the presence or absence of a sheath.

If present the shape of the sheath is also important. The intermediate host and the diurnal variation of the parasitaemia all help to confirm the diagnosis. *Wucheria bancrofti* is present in the blood at night, *Loa loa* during the day.

Pathology

A. *The Adult Worms*

Adults may lead to problems by —

(i) their physical presence — ascaris can cause intestinal obstruction, intestinal perforation and obstruction of the biliary duct.

(ii) their mode of attachment to the host and their nutrition, e.g. hookworms attach to villi in the intestine and blood flows into the intestinal lumen of the worm, much of which is secreted undigested by the worm. Hookworms move from one villus to another leaving a path of oozing villi behind them.

B. *The Larvae*

Those larvae which migrate through various of the host's organs prior to settling may present the following problems —

(*a*) They may lose their way and be trapped in a site deleterious to the host.

(*b*) During their migration they can damage tissue and evoke various host responses, e.g. dyspnoea, cough, eosinophilia.

(*c*) The host may respond to the presence of the adult worm or the larvae with a hypersensitivity type of reaction. Infection with certain of the nematodes can lead to allergic responses.

Prevention and control

Therapy is available which will kill the adult worms. If multiple worm infestation has occurred in a single individual's intestinal tract, it is advisable to treat the ascaris infection first. Ascaris is an irritable worm. Although it is unlikely to have caused the patient's symptoms it can cause serious consequences should it be irritated by treatment used to kill the other worms. An irritable ascarid is an active worm and likely to cause acute obstruction of the intestine or the bile duct.

Nematode infections that can be prevented by adequate hygiene are spread by the faecal-oral route. Hands are a major source of spread. Larvae which actively penetrate the skin usually do so at the level of the feet or ankles. They are incapable of penetrating leather, therefore boots will decrease the incidence of hookworm in endemic areas. Adequate sanitation is of course the better mode of preventing spread.

Filaria can be avoided by protecting the individual against mosquitoes, flies and midges. DDT and other insecticides are of value.

Dracunculus medinensis

The 'Guinea Worm' is of great medical interest. The female is a long worm found in skin blisters in the infected host. Treatment is removal of the worm using a matchstick. Each time the matchstick is turned, a few more millimetres of the worm are extracted from the skin. Medical associations sport dracunculus wound around a stick on their badges.

Man, the definitive host, sheds the larvae when the skin blister contacts water and bursts. Infected crustaceans, e.g. cyclops are in turn ingested by man.

Acquisition of this infestation is prevented by adequate boiling of water. Spread is intercepted by preventing those infected by dracunculus from allowing their blisters to burst in, and hence contaminate, the local wells.

THE HIGHER PROTISTS

There are two groups of higher protists that require consideration from a medical viewpoint. These are: (A) The Protozoa; (B) The Fungi.

(A) THE PROTOZOA

The most important 'medical' protozoa are found in the groupings sarcomastigophora and sporozoa. Protozoa are single celled creatures often characterized by a particular mode of transport, e.g. the flagellates have flagellae, the amoebae move by amoeboid movement. Reproduction in this group can be either sexual or asexual. Asexual reproduction can be characterized as simple binary fission — one becomes two — or multiple fission (schigony) where one becomes more than two.

THE SARCOMASTIGOPHORA

Reproduction in this group is basically asexual by binary fission. Two groups are identified: (*a*) The Flagellates; (*b*) The Amoebae.

(a) The flagellates

Gut and genito-urinary flagellates are spread by direct or indirect contact. *Trichomonas vaginalis* is an important genito-urinary flagellate. It is transmitted venereally. In the female it usually leads to pruritis and a frothy discharge. Trichomonas prefers a less acid pH than that normally found in the vagina. Alteration of hormone balance may thus be associated with an altered vaginal pH and trichomonas proliferation. The presence of this pear-shaped organism on a vaginal smear is diagnostic.

Giardia lamblia is a pathogenic gut parasite. It is diagnosed by the presence of cysts or the vegetative form in the faeces. The portal of entry is the mouth.

Blood flagellates, e.g. trypanosomes, and tissue flagellates, e.g. leishmania both require arthropod vectors. Blood and tissue flagellates go through a variety of morphological forms. They are named according to their flagellum, e.g. the amistigote form is rounded and has no flagellum visible, while the tryptomastigote form has a flagellum running the whole length of the body and protruding at the distal end. Figure 16 shows the various morphological forms assumed by trypanosomes.

TRYPOMASTIGOTE   AMASTIGOTE   EPIMASTIGOTE   PROMASTIGOTE

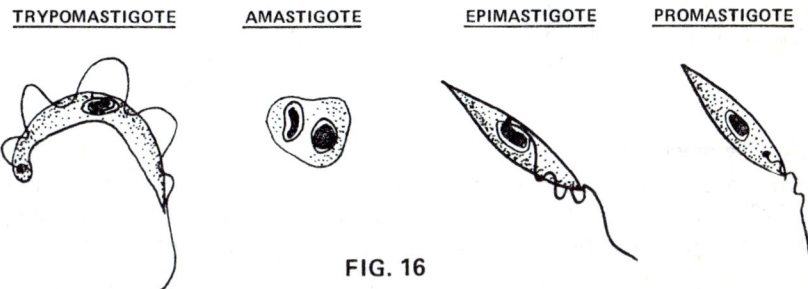

FIG. 16

In all cases a local lesion or chancre occurs at the site of the bite of the insect vector. The trypanosomes and *Leishmania donovani* do not remain localized but spread systemically. These diseases are responsible for a proportion of the morbidity and mortality associated with tropical diseases. *Trypanosoma gambiense* is responsible for a devastating disease. Sleeping sickness was recognised by the slave traders — any African who had posterior cervical lymphadenopathy was rejected as a potential slave. An early sign of sleeping sickness is lymphadenopathy, end stage sleeping sickness is manifest as emaciation, a stuporised state and later coma and death.

Trypanosomes are of interest to immunologists as they are thought capable of changing their surface antigens. In this way they continually evade the host's defences.

Control of these diseases can be achieved if the vector and/or host are separated from man. The habits of both the vector and reservoir hosts have been studied. In the past large areas were depleted of game in an effort to control trypanosomiasis. Today more conservative methods are applied, e.g. bush clearing, the sterilization of male tse-tse flies and the use of insecticides. Men who during their work or pleasure are exposed to these diseases are advised to take adequate precautions. Drug therapy is available but is itself toxic.

Table XXI
DISEASE AND THE FLAGELLATES

ORGANISM	VECTOR	RESERVOIR HOST	DISEASE IN MAN	MODE OF TRANSMISSION
BLOOD FLAGELLATES — THE TRYPANOSOMES				
T. Brucei gambiense	Glossina (tse-tse fly)	man	Sleeping sickness	bite
T. brucei rhodesiense	Glossina (tse-tse fly)	wild and domestic animals	Rhodesian trypaniso-miasis	bite
T. cruzi	Treatoma (bug)	dog, cat, monkey	Chagas disease	scratching infected faeces into skin lesion
TISSUE FLAGELLATES — LEISHMANIA				
L.donovani	Phlebotomus (sand-fly)	dog, fox, rodent	Kala-azar (Visceral Leishmaniasis)	bite
L.tropica	Phlebotomus (sand-fly)	dog, rodent	Cutaneous Leishmaniasis	bite
L.braziliensis	Phlebotomus (sand-fly)	dog	Espundia (mucocuta-neous Leish-maniasis)	bite

(b) The amoebae

Amoebae form a group of organisms some of which are parasites, others of which are free living. The different types of amoebae are identified by features characteristic of both the trophozoite and cyst forms.

Entamoeba histolytica is the invasive pathogenic amoebae responsible for amoebic dysentry and liver disease in man. It is diagnosed in the trophozoite stage by its cartwheel nucleus, the presence of ingested erythrocytes and the explosive movement of its pseudopodia. The cyst form has four nuclei and spiky chromidial bars. *Entamoeba coli* may be present as a commensal in the intestinal tract and must be distinguished from this pathogenic amoeba.

The factors which precipitate invasion by *Entamoeba histolytica* are unknown. Factors postulated to precipitate invasion include dietary changes, a mucosal lesion and subjection of the host to stress factors.

Transmission of the organism is from man to man. Faecal oral spread of cysts occurs by food contamination, e.g. the lettuce fertilized by human excreta. Trophozoites quickly succumb to environmental conditions. The cyst forms are the resistant forms. The cyst is viable after being at a temperature of 20°C for 30 days; it also resists the effects of certain disinfectants, e.g. chlorine and formalin. Storage followed by inadequate washing of infected vegetables is a common source of transmission, provided the vegetables are eaten raw.

Figure 17
THE LIFE CYCLE OF AN AMOEBA

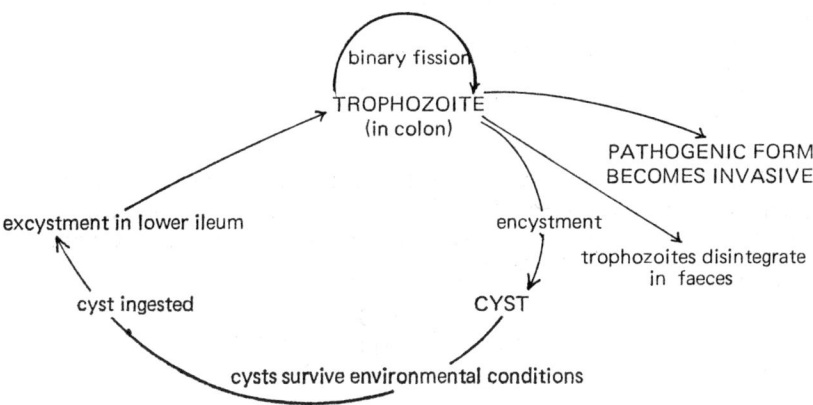

Control of amoebiasis is by adequate sanitation and good personal hygiene. Treatment is with metranidazole. This drug is also used in the treatment of *Trichomonas vaginalis* infections.

THE SPOROZOA

Important pathogens in this sub-phylum include —

> Pneumocystis
> Toxoplasma
> Plasmodium

Pneumocystis carinii is an important pathogen in patients with depressed immunity. In hosts with defective immunity, pneumocystis causes an interstitial pneumonia.

Toxoplasma gondii can be transmitted transplacentally causing congenital abnormalities in the foetus. Like rubella, primary toxoplasmosis contracted during pregnancy leads to serious foetal damage.

Toxoplasmosis may be contracted by ingestion of oocysts excreted in cat faeces. Another route of transmission is the ingestion of toxoplasmic cysts in undercooked meat, e.g. mutton. Pregnant women with negative serological tests for toxoplasma should avoid contact with cats and the eating of undercooked meat.

Toxoplasmosis is a mild, usually sub-clinical disease in the adult. Relapse of chronic toxoplasmosis can occur in patients on immunosuppression.

The plasmodia form an important group of sporozoa. These are the agents responsible for malaria. Different species of plasmodia cause different types of malaria.

Table XXII

PLASMODIA PATHOGENIC TO MAN

ORGANISM	TYPE OF DISEASE	RELAPSES	PARASITAEMIA
Plasmodium vivax	Benign tertian malaria	+	+
Plasmodium falciparum	Malignant tertian malaria	−	+++
Plasmodium malariae	Quartian malaria	++	+
Plasmodium ovale	Ovale malaria	+	+

The life cycle of the malaria parasite is complex. *Plasmodium falciparum* differs from the other forms of malaria in not causing relapses, i.e. in any one malarial infection with falciparum the organisms are only capable of one hepatic phase of development.

Figure 18
THE PLASMODIUM LIFE CYCLE

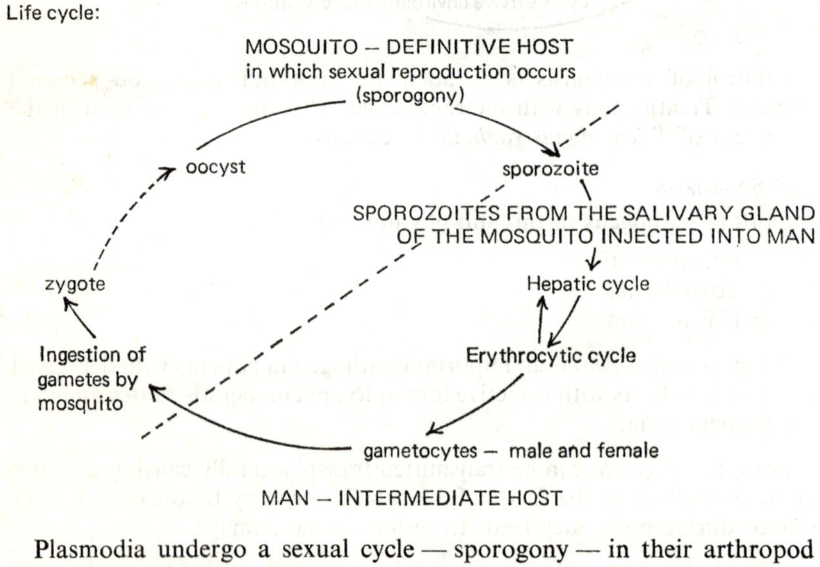

Life cycle:

MOSQUITO — DEFINITIVE HOST
in which sexual reproduction occurs
(sporogony)

oocyst   sporozoite

SPOROZOITES FROM THE SALIVARY GLAND
OF THE MOSQUITO INJECTED INTO MAN

zygote   Hepatic cycle

Ingestion of   Erythrocytic cycle
gametes by
mosquito

gametocytes — male and female

MAN — INTERMEDIATE HOST

Plasmodia undergo a sexual cycle — sporogony — in their arthropod host. Their arthropod host is the anopheles mosquito. The definitive host of plasmodia is the mosquito.

The female anophelene mosquito requires a blood meal for the normal maturation of her eggs. On biting an infected host (man) she may ingest macro (female) and micro (male) gametocytes. These gametes fuse and the sexual cycle involving a number of different morphological forms follows. The infective product of sexual reproduction is the sporozoite. Sporozoites present in the salivary glands of the female mosquito are transferred to a new host (man) when the mosquito takes her next blood meal.

Two different species of anopheles transmit plasmodia — their distribution and incidence determine whether an area will have endemic malaria or outbreaks of epidemic malaria. *Anopheles funestus* breeds in permanent shaded water and thus is always present and is associated with endemic malaria. *Anopheles gambiae* breeds in shallow open pools, e.g. cattle hoof marks filled with rain water. *Anopheles gambiae* multiply profusely during a heavy rainy season following a drought. Epidemics of malaria are thus most likely to occur during the rains following prolonged drought. Malarial outbreaks are related to the habits of the definitive host and not the organism itself.

The type of organism, i.e. the type of plasmodium, does determine the clinical disease in man. *Plasmodium falciparium* gives rise to malignant tertian malaria. This species frequently causes cerebral malaria. It causes non-relapsing malaria. *Plasmodium ovale* and *Plasmodium vivax* both produce a relatively benign disease which tends to relapse for up to 3 years after the initial infection. *Plasmodium malariae* causes benign quartian malaria which can relapse for up to 20 years after the initial attack.

Relapses are due to the ability of certain species to re-infect the host's liver during a parasitaemia. *Plasmodium falciparum*, having once passed through its hepatic phase, enters the blood and the products of schizogony are incapable of re-infecting the liver.

Acute malaria is clinically characterized by fever, rigors and sweating. Jaundice may develop. The severity of the clinical symptoms are directly related to the degree of parasitaemia. The schizogony phase of plasmodial development is directly related to lysis of the parasitized red blood cells. Anaemia is a feature of malaria.

Diagnosis of malaria depends on the examination of blood films. Species identification is possible on the morphological characteristics of the plasmodia in the blood film. The percentage of erythrocytes which are parasitized is an index of the severity of the clinical disease.

Early and adequate treatment of malaria can be life saving. Different drugs act on different stages of the organism's development. The hepatic forms of the organism are more difficult to treat and eliminate than those in the blood. Clinical cure is possible in the presence of hepatic parasites — the clinical symptoms are related to the multiplication of the parasites in erythrocytes. Radicle cure implies the death of all the plasmodia in that host.

Prophalaxis against malaria is practised for both personal and public health reasons. The individual taking anti-malarials prophalactically does so before, during and after being in a malarial area. The drugs do not prevent the organism infecting the host, they suppress the clinical symptoms of the disease. Suppressive phropalaxis should thus be taken for a

month after leaving the malarial area. Causal prophalaxis involves the use
of more toxic anti-malarials. These latter drugs are capable of interfering
with the hepatic phase of the organism's development. A good method of
preventing malaria is not to be bitten by the mosquito — mosquito nets,
sun-downers behind mesh screens and the wearing of long sleeves are all
thus of value in preventing malaria.

Public health authorities in malaria endemic areas exert some control
over this disease by attempting to control the mosquitoes. House spraying,
and nctting are measures employed against the adults; larvae are killed
by spreading layers of oil over water used by mosquitoes for breeding.
Receptive areas are those areas with mosquitoes but no malaria. A single
individual with malaria entering this area could infect the mosquito population.

(B) THE FUNGI

Fungi are higher protists with relatively rigid cell walls. They are found
in two forms —
- (*a*) as unicellular organisms — yeasts.
- (*b*) as multicellular filaments — moulds.

Aggregates of hyphae are called mycelia or moulds.

From the medical viewpoint, fungi can interact with man in a variety
of ways —
- (*a*) They can cause food poisoning, e.g. mushrooms.
- (*b*) They may be aetiologically implicated in certain carcinomas, e.g.
  primary hepatoma is linked to aflatoxin on circumstantial evidence.
- (*c*) Hypersensitivity to various fungi is well recognised, e.g. asthma due
  to aspergillus; allergic alveolitis is associated with mouldy hay
  and/or sugar cane.
- (*d*) They can cause infections.

Fungal infections are divided into two groups —
- (i) superficial;
- (ii) deep.

(i) SUPERFICIAL FUNGAL INFECTIONS

The single most important fungal infection is ringworm. Ringworm is a
fungal infection of keratin-containing structures — skin, hair and nails.
The dermatophytes are the fungi causing ringworm. There are three important genera — *Microsporum*, *Epidermophyton*, and *Trichophyton*.

These fungi may be divided into —
- (i) Anthropophilic fungi — those infecting man.
- (ii) Zoophilic fungi — ringworm usually associated with animal infections.
- (iii) Geophilic fungi — soil fungi.

Infection of man by a zoophilic or geophilic fungus results in a more marked inflammatory reaction than infection by an anthrophilic fungus.

Hair infection may lead to weakening of the hair shaft and the hair may break off close to the scalp. Certain types of ringworm can therefore cause baldness. Infected nails become brittle and lustreless. A variety of skin lesions develop.

Although localized skin ringworm is amenable to topical therapy, hair, nail or extensive skin involvement require systemic therapy. Therapy is long-term.

Ringworm of different anatomical areas has acquired a variety of different names — Tinea pedis — 'Athletes' foot'.
Tinea capitis — ringworm of the scalp.
Tinea corporis — body ringworm, etc.

Ringworm is the only fungal disease readily transmitted from man to man.

(ii) THE DEEP MYCOSES
Many of the fungi capable of causing a deep fungal infection are found in the environment. Certain fungi cause primary infection, others are responsible for secondary or opportunistic infections.

A large number of fungi breach the skin barrier of the host, and often they are introduced into a traumatized area of skin. Lesions caused by this group of fungi usually have a primary skin or subcutaneous lesion. Clinically, ulcers or sinuses are invariably present. Blastomycosis, sporotrichosis, chromomycosis, phycomycosis and mycetoma are all examples of this type of infection.

Mycetoma is a subcutaneous mycosis caused by two different groups of organisms — one group of organisms causing this disease are true fungi, the other group are members of the actinomycetes. Actinomycetes respond to antibiotic and not to antifungal therapy.

A second group of fungi are inhaled and may cause primary lung pathology. Fungal infection of the lung may range from a diffuse infiltration to a single tumour-like mass. Cryptococcosis can present in the lung as a mass or in the brain as a cause of raised intra-cranial pressure. Both histoplasmosis and coccidiomycosis give rise to a benign 'flue-like' illness. Dissemination of histoplasmosis to the reticulo-endothelial system is rare but fatal. When coccidiodomycosis disseminates to skin, bones, the central nervous system and other organs, it is fatal. All the deep mycoses mentioned are associated with environmental contact with the organism — many of these fungi are found in soil, wood or plant matter. These infections are exogenous infections.

Endogenous infections may be caused by *Actinomycetes israelii* or *Candida albicans*. *Actinomycetes israelii* is a normal inhabitant of the mouth.

The organism is not contagious and disease results from endogenous infection of traumatised mucous membrane. Actinomycotic lesions are found mainly in one of three sites — cervico-facial, abdominal or thoracic. Treatment is with penicillin. Actinomycosis is not caused by a true fungus.

Candida albicans is a true fungus found as a commensal in the mouth and intestinal tract. Endogenous infection is especially common in the very young, the very old, the diabetic, in people on antibiotics — especially those on broad spectrum antibiotics which interfere with the normal flora, and in macerated areas, e.g. in areas traumatised due to prolonged skin wetness. Candida can infect nails, the skin and mucous membranes of the mouth and genitalia. It can also spread systemically. The classical candida lesion on mucous membranes is the white patch; on skin a variety of different 'patches' are found. Candida is a fungus capable of causing disease in apparently healthy people as well as in certain individuals with a defect in their host defences. Other fungal diseases found in individuals with defective host defences are aspergillosis and phycomycosis. Spread of candida in hospitals is rarely due to cross-infection. Aspergillosis and phycomycosis are exogenous infections and their spread in hospitals may be as a result of environmental contamination or by cross-infection.

Aspergillus fumigatus can be a secondary invader in lungs with impaired defences due to damage by tuberculosis, asbestosis or sarcoidosis. This fungus can exist as a saphrophyte in old tuberculous cavities. It may, however, produce an allergic alveolitis or become invasive. The incidence of metastasis of aspergillus to the brain and other organs is highest in individuals suffering from haematological disorders.

Phycomycosis is caused by fungi which live saprophytically on decaying vegetable matter. Diabetics and leukaemics are especially prone to infections of the sinuses with this organism. The fungus invades locally, spreading to the brain. Unless early and adequate treatment is started, this condition is rapidly fatal.

Table XXIII

POTENTIALLY PATHOGENIC ENVIRONMENTAL FUNGI

FUNGI FOUND IN THE SOIL	PRIMARY CLINICAL LESION
Aspergillus	Lung lesion, allergic, disseminated
Cryptococcus	Pulmonary lesion, meningitis
Blastomycetes	Skin lesion
Histoplasma	Skin or pulmonary lesions
Coccidiodes	Respiratory infection
Paracoccidiodes	Muco-cutaneous
Geophilic ringworm	Skin
FUNGI FOUND ASSOCIATED WITH WOOD/PLANT MATTER	
Phialophora (causes Chromomycosis)	Skin
Sporothrix	Skin

The host's response to fungal infections is usually determined by the efficiency of his cell mediated immunity.

Granulomatous lesions form the common type of histological picture. The fungi can appear as yeasts or mycelia. Certain fungi are dimorphic, i.e. they are yeast-like at 37,5°C (body temperature) and therefore yeast-like in tissue sections; at room temperature they, however, revert to their filamentous form.

Diagnosis of fungal infections are made by —

(i) direct examination of tissue sections, scrapings or excreta;
(ii) culture.

Treatment of fungal infections is occasionally surgical but usually involves the use of anti-fungal agents. The standard anti-fungal agents for topical use include desquamating agents. Those for systemic use include griseofulvin and amphotericin B. The anti-mitotic agent, 5-fluoro cytosine, and iodides have been used in the successful treatment of certain fungal conditions. Fungi and man have in common a eukaryotic cell type. Anti-fungal agents are thus more toxic to the host than anti-bacterial agents. Clinical cure often precedes mycological cure and therefore treatment must not be discontinued as soon as the patient feels better.

Fungi are widely distributed in nature. Environmental fungi assume new importance in medicine in an age where immunosuppression is widely used. The incidence of serious fungal infections is increasing in direct proportion to the increase in the use of immunosuppressives.

BACTERIA

A large number of bacteria do not cause disease. Some live in dead organic matter and are called saprophytes. Saprophytes are important in industrial and agricultural microbiology. Saprophytes are responsible for the ripening of cheese, the fermentation of carbohydrate leading to alcohol production and the acidification of milk. In nature bacteria are involved in carbon, nitrogen and sulphur cycles. Decomposition of organic matter is thus associated with the action of bacteria. Those bacteria which do cause disease fall into two groups:

A. THE PATHOGENS

These are capable of causing disease because they are endowed with special properties. Pathogens may be arbitrarily placed in one of two groups depending on their clinical presentation —

(*a*) Those which give rise to specific syndromes, e.g. typhoid, tetanus.
(*b*) Those which, in common with other organisms, cause a syndrome dependent on the organ of the host which is involved, e.g. meningitis, gastro-enteritis.

B. THE OPPORTUNISTS

These organisms may be saprophytes, which on being removed from their normal environment and introduced into certain susceptible hosts, cause disease. The disease pattern in such cases is less related to the organism's ability to cause disease than the inability of the host to defend himself.

Opportunistic pathogens may also be grouped as commensals. Commensals are organisms usually found in certain sites of the body. They do no harm in their natural habitat, e.g. *Streptococcus viridans* in the throat, *Staphylococcus epidermidis* on the skin. If either of these organisms is introduced into an unusual anatomical site, e.g. a heart valve, they become opportunistic pathogens and cause disease.

CLASSIFICATION

Table XXIV
BACTERIA OF MEDICAL IMPORTANCE

GROUPINGS BASED ON THE GRAM STAIN AND MORPHOLOGY — A LIGHT MICROSCOPIC CLASSIFICATION

GENUS	SPECIES	IMPORTANT CAUSES OF
GRAM-POSITIVE COCCI		
STREPTOCOCCUS	*Streptococcus pyogenes*	Throat and skin infection (N.B. delayed sequelae)
	Streptococcus pneumoniae	Pneumonia, meningitis
	Streptococcus mutans	Dental caries
	Streptococcus faecalis	Opportunists — urinary tract infection, bacterial endocarditis
	Streptococcus viridans	Endocarditis

Standard culture media — Blood agar, Nutrient agar.
Selective media — MacConkey, aesculin bile.

STAPHYLOCOCCUS	*Staphylococcus aureus* (*Staphylococcus pyogenes*)	Localized suppuration, food poisoning, septicaemia
	Staphylococcus epidermidis	Opportunists — bacterial endocarditis

Standard culture media — Blood agar.
Selective media — Chapman's agar (high salt content).

GRAM-NEGATIVE COCCI		
NEISSERIA (diplococci)	*Neisseria gonorrhoeae*	Gonorrhoea
	Neisseria meningitidis	Meningitis

Standard culture media — Chocolate agar (5-10% CO_2).
Selective media — Thayer-Martin (above plus antibiotics).

GRAM-POSITIVE BACILLI		
LACTOBACILLUS	*Lactobacillus acidophilus*	Responsible for acid pH in mature vagina

Selective media — Tomato agar.

CORYNEBACTERIUM	*Corynebacterium diphtheriae*	Diphtheria

Standard media — Blood Agar.
Selective media — Hoyles plate (Potassium tellurite), Loefflers slope.

BACILLUS	*Bacillus anthracis*	Anthrax
CLOSTRIDIUM	*Clostridium tetani*	Tetanus
	Clostridium botulinum	Botulism
	Clostridium perfringens *Clostridium novyi* *Clostridium septicum*	Gas gangrene

Selective culture media — Willis and Hobbs plate.

GENUS	SPECIES	IMPORTANT CAUSES OF

GRAM-NEGATIVE BACILLI
A. SMALL GRAM-NEGATIVE BACILLI/PARVOBACTERIA

BRUCELLA — *Brucella abortus* / *Brucella melitensis* / *Brucella suis* — Brucellosis

Selective media — Castenedas medium

HAEMOPHILUS — *Haemophilus influenzae* — Meningitis, respiratory tract infections

Haemophilus aegypticus — Conjunctivitis

Selective media — BHB (Bacitracin in haemolysed blood).

BORDATELLA — *Bordatella pertussis* — Whooping cough

Selective medium — Bordet-Gengou medium

YERSINIA — *Yersinia pestis* — Plague — bubonic, pneumonic, septicaemic

Yersinia enterocolitica — Arthritis, mesenteric adenitis, gastro-enteritis

PASTURELLA — *Pasturella multocida* — Abscess (zoonosis)

BACTEROIDES — *Bacteroides fragilis* — Abscess (anaerobic conditions)

B. THE ENTEROBACTERIACEAE

SALMONELLA — *Salmonella typhi* — Typhoid

Salmonella species — Gastro-enteritis

SHIGELLA — *Shigella dysenteriae* / *Shigella sonnei* / *Shigella flexneri* / *Shigella boydii* — Bacillary dysentry

Selective media — S.S. medium (Shigella — Salmonella medium).

ESCHERICHIA — *Escherichia coli* — Opportunist — urinary tract infection, neonatal meningitis, infant diarrhoea

KLEBSIELLA — *Klebsiella pneumoniae* — Pneumonia, opportunist — urinary tract infection

PROTEUS — *Proteus morgani* / *Proteus rettgeri* / *Proteus vulgaris* / *Proteus mirabilis* — Urinary tract infection — Opportunists

ENTEROBACTER, CITROBACTER, ERWINIA, PROVIDENTIA — All may cause opportunistic infection.

C. VIBRIOS

VIBRIO — *Vibrio cholerae* — Cholera

Vibrio parahaemolyticus — Food poisoning/gastro-enteritis

Selective media — T.C.B.S. (sucrose bile salt media; alkaline with an indicator).

D. PSEUDOMONAS

PSEUDOMONAS — *Pseudomonas aeruginosa* — Opportunist — wound and burns infected, septecaemia

Standard media for Gram-negative Bacilli — MacConkey.

FILAMENTOUS BACTERIA

ANAEROBIC ACTINOMYCES (gram positive) — *Actinomyces israelii* — Actinomycosis

AEROBIC NOCARDIA — *Nocardia asteroides* — Nocardiosis, Actinomycetoma

GENUS	SPECIES	IMPORTANT CAUSES OF

STRICT ANAEROBES

GRAM-NEGATIVE BACILLI — Bacteroides   Abscess, ulceration
     e.g. *Bacteroides fragilis,*
     Bacteroides melaninogenicus
     — Fusobacterium   Abscess
     e.g. *Fusobacterium nucleatum*
GRAM-POSITIVE BACILLI — Clostridia   See page 86
GRAM-POSITIVE COCCI   — Peptococci
     — Peptostreptococci   } Suppurative lesions

GROUPING BASED ON THE ZIEHL-NEELSEN STAIN AND MORPHOLOGY — ACID-FAST BACILLI

GENUS	SPECIES	IMPORTANT CAUSE OF
MYCOBACTERIUM	*M. tuberculosis*	Human tuberculosis
	M. bovis	Cattle tuberculosis (Intestinal tuberculosis in man)
	M. leprae	Leprosy

Mycobacteria not causing tuberculosis previously called atypical mycobacteria — opportunist infections, saphrophytes.
Selective media — Lowenstein Jensen.
Mycobacterium leprae does not grow on artificial culture media.

NOCARDIA	*Nocardia asteroides*	Mycetoma, Nocardiosis

A modified stain is required to demonstrate acid fastness in this aerobic actinomycete.

GROUPING BASED ON MORPHOLOGY AND DARK FIELD MICROSCOPY — SPIROCHAETES/SPIRAL ORGANISMS

GENUS	SPECIES	IMPORTANT CAUSE OF
TREPONEMA	*Treponema pallidum*	Syphilis
BORRELIA	*Borrelia recurrentis*	Relapsing fever
	Borrelia duttoni	Relapsing fever
	Borrelia vincenti	Vincent's angina (when with a fusiform bacterium)
LEPTOSPIRA	*L. icterohaemorrhagica*	Leptospirosis

Culture — highly selective, Treponemes fail to grow in artificial culture media.

The preceding organisms may be further grouped according to —

  (i) optimal growth temperature — see Table XXV. Organisms grow best at certain temperatures. Three groups of organisms have been identified on the basis of their ability to grow at certain temperatures.

  (ii) oxygen requirements — see Table XXVI. Hydrogen acceptors are substances capable of accepting a hydrogen ion during oxidation-reduction reactions. Oxidation-reduction reactions are energy yielding.

Table XXV
GROUPING OF ORGANISMS ON THE BASIS OF TEMPERATURE

BACTERIAL GROUP	TEMPERATURE RANGE FOR OPTIMAL GROWTH
PSYCHROPHILIC	15 to 20°C
MESOPHILIC	30 to 37°C
THERMOPHILIC	50 to 60°C

Bacteria pathogenic to man are usually mesophilic.

Table XXVI
ORGANISMS AS GROUPED ON THE BASIS OF THEIR RESPONSE TO OXYGEN

BACTERIAL GROUP	RELATIONSHIP TO OXYGEN
OBLIGATE AEROBE	This group specifically requires oxygen as the hydrogen acceptor. These bacteria obtain energy from respiration.
FACULTATIVE	These organisms may live in the presence or absence of oxygen. They are capable of respiration and fermentation depending on the environment.
OBLIGATE ANAEROBE	Oxygen is toxic to these bacteria. It is never used as a hydrogen acceptor by this group. These bacteria use fermentation to obtain their energy.

Bacteria pathogenic to man may fall into any one of these groups.

COCCI

Cocci are —

   (i) spherical

  (ii) non-motile

 (iii) non-sporing

 (iv) organisms which multiply by binary fission

  (v) lower protists and bacteria.

STREPTOCOCCI

Streptococci are —

(1) Cocci in chains

(2) Gram-positive

(3) Capable of causing haemolysis — streptococci secrete enzymes, streptolysin O and S. Both these streptolysins are capable of causing damage to the cell membrane of erythrocytes. Haemolysis is tested by culturing the organisms on a blood agar plate. The resulting haemolysis may be classified as one of the following types —

α haemolysis — incomplete haemolysis resulting in a greenish zone around the colony.

β haemolysis — complete haemolysis resulting in a colourless zone around the colony.

γ haemolysis — here no haemolysis is visible (haemolysis may be detected underneath the colony).

(4)   Groups according to Lancefield's grouping — this classification of streptococci is based on the specific antigenic structure of the grouped carbohydrate. Each different type is designated with a letter from the alphabet, e.g. A, B, etc.

Figure 19

THE STRUCTURE OF A STREPTOCOCCUS

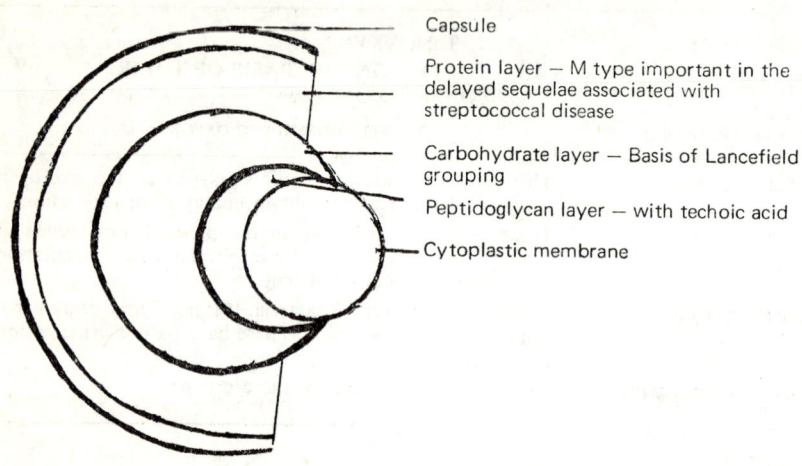

Capsule

Protein layer — M type important in the delayed sequelae associated with streptococcal disease

Carbohydrate layer — Basis of Lancefield grouping

Peptidoglycan layer — with techoic acid

Cytoplastic membrane

Streptococcus pyogenes — Beta-Haemolytic Streptococcus Group A Gram-positive cocci in chains.

Source: Patient or carrier. *Streptococcus pyogenes* may be carried by 5-10% of people. The highest carrier rate is in children. The organism may be carried on the skin or in the nose or throat.

Spread: Spread occurs by droplet spray, e.g. coughing, sneezing, or by direct contact. Transfer of the organism may be direct or by contamination of fomites such as clothing, bedding, books. The throat provides the best source of pathogenic bacteria; the nose is a better organ for the dissemination of bacteria.

Streptococci succumb to direct sunlight but can survive for weeks in dusty crevices. The main route of spread is that of close person-to-person contact permitting the spread of moist secretions.

Virulence: *Streptococcus pyogenes* causes disease in the host by its ability to —

(i)   Resist phagocytosis. Incorporated into the bacterial cell wall is a protein layer — type M protein is resistant to phagocytosis.

(ii)   Secrete a number of enzymes and toxins. Examples of these include — hyaluronidase which breaks down the ground substance of the host; streptodornase (DNAse) which depolymerises DNA and streptolysin which is toxic to host cells. A toxin which deserves special mention is erythrogenic toxin. Infection of *Streptococcus pyogenes* by a specific bacteriophage (bacterial virus) confers on this bacterium the ability to produce erythrogenic toxin. This toxin is responsible for the characteristic erythematous rash of scarlet fever.

Host: Overcrowding increases close contact and this is a major factor in the spread and incidence of streptococcal disease.

The immune response of the host to the organism can lead to delayed sequelae becoming apparent in the host some weeks after the initial infection. A decrease in the host's immunity may alter the local manifestations of the disease, e.g. a viral infection of the respiratory system may be complicated by streptococcal pneumonia.

Disease pattern: This is determined by the portal of entry of the organism. Entry by the respiratory tract is associated with a sore throat, direct contact or spread by way of a skin defect is associated with erysipelas, impetigo or another skin infection.

In a certain group of hosts, selected on the basis of their immune systems, delayed sequelae may follow *Streptococcus pyogenes* infection. These immunological complications follow some 2-4 weeks after the initial acute infection. In these individuals a sore throat may be the introduction to rheumatic fever. Many different types of *Streptococcus pyogenes* are capable of causing rheumatic fever in susceptible hosts. Contact with the organism is inevitable owing to it being widespread. A patient who has suffered one attack of rheumatic fever is therefore at risk of further attacks. With each attack of rheumatic fever the heart valves may be damaged. The patient is thus likely to suffer, at some stage of his life, haemodynamic difficulties and infection of the damaged valves (sub-acute bacterial endocarditis). The aim is thus prevention of rheumatic fever. After one attack of rheumatic fever an individual is labelled as being at risk of future attacks. These individuals must be protected against *Streptococcus pyogenes* infections. This can be achieved by the daily administration of a low dose of penicillin.

Attacks of acute glomerulonephritis may follow either skin or throat infections by *Streptococcus pyogenes*. The number of *Streptococcus pyogenes* capable of inducing renal sequelae is limited. After one attack of acute glomerulonephritis the patient is therefore not subject to years of antibiotic therapy. Eradication of the nephritogenic strain of *Streptococcus pyogenes* from the family unit is advocated. This is achieved by antibiotic therapy.

Drug of Choice: *Streptococcus pyogenes* is exquisitely sensitive to penicillin. The drug of choice in the treatment and prophylaxis of diseases caused by this organism is therefore clear cut.

Streptococcus agalactiae — Beta Haemolytic Streptococcus Group B.
Streptococcus agalactiae is found as a normal commensal in the genital tract of some 50% of females tested. This organism does the host (mother)

no harm but certain members of this group of organisms are capable of causing meningitis and septicaemia in the newborn. The organism is spread by aspiration as the baby passes through the birth canal. Premature infants and those subject to instrument delivery or prolonged labour are particularly susceptible to infection by *Streptococcus agalactiae*. *Streptococcus agalactiae* septicaemia has a 50% mortality rate.

Babies born after prolonged labour or following premature rupture of membranes are frequently given prophylactic antibiotics. In mothers who have already lost one baby due to infection with this organism, caesarian section is often considered for the delivery of the next child.

Streptococcus faecalis — Enterococci
The haemolysis of these streptococci is variable.
Source: *Streptococcus faecalis* is a natural inhabitant of the intestinal tract.

Spread: Usually by direct contact.

Virulence: They cause opportunistic infections, i.e. these organisms only cause disease when introduced into an unusual anatomical site. Transfer of the organism from the bowel to the bladder results in a urinary tract infection; transfer from the bowel to the blood stream in the presence of a deformed or damaged heart valve can lead to bacterial endocarditis.

Enterococci are responsible for a large number of endogenous infections.
Treatment: Ampicillin is the drug of choice.

Streptococcus viridans
This group of organisms gives rise to alpha haemolysis.
Source: These are oral commensals. They help to make up the salivary complement of bacteria. Saliva contains of the order of 10^9 organisms per millilitre.

Spread: They may spread by direct contact. Infections are, however, usually endogenous.

Virulence: These organisms are not primarily pathogens. They take advantage of a host's impaired immune response. They cause endogenous infections, e.g. bacteria are shed into the blood stream each time dental manipulations are performed. Sub-acute bacterial endocarditis, i.e. infection of a damaged or defective heart valve is most commonly caused by a member of the *Streptococcus viridans* group of organisms.

Of this group of organisms, *Streptococcus mutans* is the main culprit in the pathogenesis of dental caries and periodontal disease. This organism plays a role in the development of dental caries by causing a change in the environment of the tooth. Dental plaques are composed of bacteria and their products — *Streptococcus mutans* plays an important role in the formation of the plaque.

The Prevention of Endocarditis

Bacterial endocarditis caused in the presence of bacteraemia following dental manipulation can be prevented in known rheumatic fever cases. Prophylactic antibiotics can be administered just prior to the visit to the dentist. High doses of penicillin are given prior to dental manipulation in these patients. This leads to high antibiotic blood levels which kill the organism without giving it an opportunity to establish itself on the distorted valve. Therapy for the prevention of sub-acute bacterial endocarditis caused by *Streptococcus viridans* is penicillin given in high doses for a limited period.

Treatment: *Streptococcus viridans* is sensitive to penicillin. It is, however, much less sensitive than *Streptococcus pyogenes*. Prophylaxis against rheumatic fever and sub-acute bacterial endocarditis differs — the type of antibiotic used in the same, the dose vastly different.

Streptococcus pneumoniae — Pneumococci

This is the second alpha haemolytic streptococcus of importance to man.

Source: Some 30% of healthy people carry pneumococci in their throats. The organism is relatively resistant to drying and spread can therefore be in secretions — nasal or oral. Fomites and dust may harbour viable pneumococci.

Disease Pattern: There are basically two groups of pneumococci —

(*a*)   Those that are essentially commensals causing disease only if aided by some decrease in the host's resistance, e.g. a preceding viral infection, smoking or atmospheric pollution. These factors stimulate excess secretion in the respiratory tract and hence interfere with surface phagocytosis of the organism. Depression of the cough reflex, e.g. in anaesthetised or intoxicated individuals, may result in aspiration of respiratory secretions. These secretions may contain pneumococci.

This group of pneumococci takes advantage of any breach in the host's defences. They cause endogenous infections especially at the extremes of life.

(*b*)   Those pneumococci which are overtly pathogenic causing disease in primarily healthy individuals. These are exogenous infections.

The types of disease caused by pneumococci are referable to both upper and lower respiratory tracts, e.g. otitis media, sinusitis, pneumonia. Meningitis caused by pneumococci is frequently associated with a fractured base of skull. This may possibly represent spread of commensal nasopharyngeal pneumococci to the meninges.

Virulence: The organism depends for its virulence on its capsule. Pneumococci are lanceolate diplococci surrounded by a capsule. The mechanism whereby the capsule protects the organism against phagocytosis is disputed. The lipid-containing membrane of the pseudopodia may be electrically repelled by the charge on the hydrated capsule. This charge could conceivably be neutralized by opsonin or specific antibody.

There are over 80 different antigen capsular types amongst the pneumococci.

Treatment: Pneumococci are sensitive to penicillin.

Prevention: Theoretically protection against this organism could be achieved by immunization. The host produces antibodies against the capsule. Unfortunately the number of different capsular types possessed by this group of organisms makes it difficult to produce a comprehensive vaccine.

STAPHYLOCOCCI

These gram positive cocci are characteristically found in clusters.

Staphylococcus aureus

Source: Staphylococci are found in the environment. They do not necessarily multiply in the environment but may remain dormant for several months. They do multiply in moist nutrient material, e.g. milk, meat. Staphylococci are killed by moist heat; exposure to 65°C kills these organisms in 30 minutes.

Spread of staphylococci is by contact — direct or indirect, and by dust or droplet spray. Nasal, throat and skin carriage occurs.

Virulence: The infective dose of staphylococci is of the order of one million organisms. If the host's defences are compromised due to the presence of a foreign body, the infective dose drops to approximately one hundred organisms. *Staphylococcus aureus* is quick to take advantage of impaired host resistance. Hospital patients especially at risk of staphylococcal infections are the neonate, the post-operative patient, the diabetic and any individual who is elderly or debilitated.

Staphylococcus aureus depends for its virulence on the following factors:

(a)   Certain antiphagocytic properties are demonstrated by these organisms. A limited number of staphylococci have the ability to resist digestion once inside the phagocyte.

(b)   The secretion of toxins and enzymes. These toxins include enzymes which may damage cell membrane, e.g. leucocidins and haemolysins. Enterotoxin is a potent exotoxin. Enterotoxin is secreted by staphylococci which have undergone lysogenic conversion by a temperate phage, i.e. the bacterium is infected by a non-lytic bacterial virus.

Disease pattern: The diseases caused by *Staphylococcus aureus* fall into three distinct groups —

(i) Local suppuration — the pus can be found superficially, e.g. as a pustule; or subcutaneously as an abscess or carbuncle or even within organs, e.g. osteomyelitis. Infection of wounds by staphylococci can lead to wound breakdown and failure of healing. Deep infections with staphylococci which may assure importance are pneumonia, a perinephric abscess and septicaemia.

(ii) Food poisoning — this is an intoxication and not an infection. The food, often meat, is contaminated — usually at some stage of processing. The staphylococci can be introduced on the fingers of the housewife or other foodhandler. Foodhandlers should not be carriers of staphylococci. The organism multiplies in the food, producing its toxin. Ideal conditions for multiplication are warmth and moisture. If the meat is heated, in other words if the meat is subject to temperatures of over 65°C for over half an hour, the organisms will be killed but the enterotoxin will not be inactivated. Enterotoxin is heat stable, its action will be unaffected even after temperatures reaching 100°C have been maintained for three minutes. Persons subsequently eating the meat ingest toxin and not viable organisms. Enterotoxin causes vomiting, and sometimes diarrhoea, 2-8 hours after its ingestion.

(iii) Staphylococcal enterocolitis — this infection may be fatal. It is a result of interference with the normal microbial flora. The normal microbial flora may be depleted due to the administration of a broad spectrum antibiotic. *Staphylococcus aureus*, if resistant to this antibiotic, proliferates and causes disease.

Staphylococci in the Hospital

Staphylococci are important in the hospital situation where they are associated with antibiotic resistance. These organisms are capable of incorporating pieces of genetic material called plasmids. The plasmid may confer certain new properties on the organism, e.g. the ability to resist antibiotics. Immunity to antibiotics may be conferred on the organism by giving it the ability to produce enzymes capable of breaking down the antibiotic, e.g. penicillinase may be introduced. Organisms containing plasmids which confer resistance to certain antibiotics will thus be favoured in hospital situations where frequent exposure to those antibiotics is possible. The organism resistant to the antibiotic has an advantage over the organism which is sensitive. In an antibiotic environment selective pressure is then placed on the microbial population. Hospital environments select strains of staphylococci for hospital or antibiotic. Community staphylococci are frequently successfully treated with penicillin, hospital acquired staphylococci are usually resistant to this antibiotic. Hospital staphylococci constitute an antibiotic resistant population.

Staphylococcus epidermidis

Source: This organism is a normal skin commensal.

Spread: *Staphylococcus epidermidis* is only pathogenic if transferred to an area of the body which is normally sterile. It causes endogenous infections.

Disease Pattern: Infection of damaged heart valves leads to sub-acute bacterial endocarditis. *Staphylococcus epidermidis* may have a rôle in the pathogenesis of acne.

Treatment: This organism is often more resistant to antimicrobial therapy than is *Staphylococcus pyogenes*.

NEISSERIA

Some characteristics of this group —
   (i) They are Gram-negative cocci.
   (ii) The pathogens present as kidney bean-shaped diplococci.
   (iii) Their natural host is man.
   (iv) They are very sensitive to environmental conditions.

Neisseria meningitidis

Source: Five to thirty per cent of the population carries *Neisseria meningitidis* in their throats. During epidemics this carrier rate reaches 80% and over. The only natural host for the organism is man.

Spread: Spread of *N. meningitidis* is person to person. The main danger of acquiring the organism is from carriers rather than cases. As the organism is very sensitive to sunlight and drying, spread requires close contact. Overcrowding leads to a three-fold increase in the carrier rate.

Virulence: *N. meningitidis* usually causes disease in a host who has some defect in his immunity — this defect is often of a transient nature, e.g. following a viral infection. Neisseria resist phagocytosis due to the presence of a capsule. They are Gram-negative organisms and therefore have endotoxin or lipopolysaccharide incorporated in their cell walls. Endotoxin is released on lysis of the bacteria.

Disease Pattern: Meningococcal meningitis is a well recognised entity. Meningitis due to this organism peaks around late winter and early spring. The seasonal fluctuation of meningococcal meningitis is well recognised. Meningoccocaemia or meningococcal septicaemia is a condition which may be fulminating. The overall mortality rate for meningococcal disease is 5-10%.

Treatment: Meningococci are becoming increasingly resistant to sulphonamides. Today the treatment of choice for meningococcal meningitis is no longer sulphonamides but penicillin.

Prevention and Prophylaxis

Neisseria meningitidis has a polysaccharide capsule which is antigenic. The antigenic constituents determine if the organism is Type A, B or C, or one of those less frequently encountered in the clinical situation. Vaccines containing extracts from *N. meningitidis* types A and C are available for persons at risk.

Individuals who have been in contact with a case of meningococcal meningitis may elect to be placed on prophylactic antimicrobial therapy. Rifampicin and minocycline are used. Certain authorities advocate careful observation in the absence of prophylaxis, others feel that prophylaxis will decrease further spread of the organism.

Neisseria gonorrhoeae

Source: The genital tract of man.

Spread: Venereal. These organisms are extremely sensitive to ultra-violet light, to dessication and also to disinfectants. Toilet seats are an unlikely mode of spread. Spread is by direct intimate person-to-person contact.

Virulence: Gonococci colonize a new host by attaching to the superficial cells of mucous membranes. Stratified squamous epithelium is relatively resistant to penetration by gonococci. The gonococci attach to the cells of the mucous membrane by means of pili. Pili are protuberances extending from the cytoplasmic membrane of the organism. For gonococci to be infective they require the presence of these thin needle-like pili. Gonococci left on a shaded cool wooden toilet seat for a few hours remain viable but are not infective as they have lost their pili. Gonococci once attached to the host's cells via the pili are rendered relatively resistant to phagocytosis.

Disease Pattern: Gonorrhoea usually symptomatic in males is often asymptomatic in females. It is a medical and social problem. In certain countries gonorrhoea is second only to the common cold in incidence. Systemic spread of the organism can result in gonococcal septicaemia — this may be acute or chronic. Gonococcal arthritis, salpingitis, proctitis and asymptomatic pharyngitis are but a few of the conditions attributed to this organism.

An infant passing through an infected birth canal can acquire a gonococcal infection of the eye. Opthalmia neonatorum can lead to blindness.

Treatment: Penicillin is the drug of choice. Some strains of gonococci have recently been reported as having developed resistance to this organism.

At birth silver nitrate or penicillin drops are routinely instilled into the eyes of the newborn. This is a precaution against an asymptomatic mother infecting her baby.

BACILLI

Bacilli are —

  (i) rod-shaped organisms;

  (ii) classified as bacteria amongst the lower protists;

  (iii) capable of being classified into broad groups on the basis of their morphology and staining reactions using either the Gram or the

Ziehl-Neelsen stain. They may be further classified on the basis of their ability to excrete certain potent exotoxins or on their characteristic metabolic profile.

(vi) They multiply by binary fission.

GRAM-POSITIVE BACILLI

Certain Gram-positive bacilli are capable of producing spores. A major division in this group is thus into spore forming organisms and non-sporing organisms. Certain vegetative cells may under adverse environmental conditions undergo a physical change and develop spores. Sporulation results in the production of the spore form of the organism which is resistant to heat, cold, dessication and disinfectants. The spore is essentially a resting stage. It is a resistant but non-reproductive form of the organism. When conditions become favourable, e.g. adequate moisture becomes available, the spore may germinate and revert to the vegetative form. The vegetative form of the bacillus is capable of multiplication or binary fission.

Spore forms are resistant to temperature and disinfectants and therefore constitute a problem in the hospital environment. Minimal requirements for sterility are determined by the resistance of spores to heat. Temperature and exposure time are determined by the ability of the spore to resist death. Spores of *Bacillus stearothermophilus* are used as a biological sterility control. The spores of this non-pathogenic organism are placed in a packet and introduced into the autoclave in the centre of the pack to be sterilized. After autoclaving an attempt is made to culture the organism. If the spores fail to germinate under favourable conditions then the spores are dead and it may be assumed that the pack is sterile. This biological control, in conjunction with steritape, is routinely used in hospitals. Both saprophytes and pathogens are found amongst Gram-positive bacilli.

Spore forming Gram-positive bacilli

This group of organisms is further divided into aerobic and anaerobic groups.

Aerobic spore forming Gram-positive bacilli

Bacillus stearothermophilus

A saprophyte used as the biological control for sterility testing of autoclaved material.

Bacillus anthracis

Bacillus anthracis causes anthrax. Anthrax is a zoonosis, i.e. it is a disease spread from animals to man.

Source: Certain population groups are at risk of exposure to anthrax. *Bacillus anthracis* may cause a fatal disease in sheep, cattle and horses. People at risk are those working with animal hides, the wool sorters and those working with animal carcasses.

Spread: The organism may be inhaled, ingested or may be spread to a new host by contact with a skin lesion. *B. anthracis* is usually spread in the spore form.

Virulence: The spore germinates at its site of entry. *B. anthracis* is pathogenic due to —

(a) The presence of a capsule. This capsule is composed of polypeptide units. Most organisms with capsules have polysaccharide capsules. Notable exceptions are *Yersinia pestis* and *B. anthracis* with their polypeptide capsule. On culture these colonies are said to have a 'Medusa head' appearance.

(b) Its ability to produce toxins. Three heat sensitive substances are produced. These substances are called fractions 1, 2 and 3. Fraction 1, the oedema factor and fraction 3, the lethal factor are required together with fraction 2 for efficient pathogenicity. Fraction 2, the protective factor, is antigenic and it is against this fraction that the host produces antibody.

Disease Pattern: The clinical picture of anthrax is largely determined by its portal of entry. Entry of the organism into a skin lesion results in formation of a malignant pustule; inhalation results in haemorrhagic mediastinitis and ingestion of poorly cooked meat results in intestinal anthrax.

Treatment: Penicillin is the drug of choice. Anthrax may be fatal.

Prevention and Control: Anthrax is primarily a disease of animals and the control of this problem rests essentially at this level. Cattle and sheep should be immunized against the disease. The live vaccine is too toxic for use in man. Men at risk of exposure to anthrax are protected by a fraction 2 antigen vaccine. Frequent boosters are required. Men working with animals in an anthrax endemic area are obliged to wear protective clothing.

Animals dying of suspected anthrax are incinerated or buried in deep lime (anaerobic conditions inhibit spore formation). Post mortems are not performed, but a splenic aspirate may be performed. These precautions decrease the probability of spore formation. Anthrax spores are known to have survived for over 100 years.

Bacillus cereus

Source: The organism is thought to grow on rice and other cereals.

Virulence: A toxin is produced.

Disease Pattern: The toxin produced induces vomiting. The gastroenteritis caused by *Bacillus cereus* is characterised by the onset of symptoms within two hours after ingestion of the infected food.

Anaerobic spore forming Gram-positive bacilli

The important pathogens in this group are the clostridia.

Source: Clostridia are found in soil. They are also normal inhabitants of the gastrointestinal tract of both man and animals. Exposure to clostridia is inevitable. Infection may be endogenous or exogenous.

Virulence: Clostridia cause disease by secretion of exotoxins. It is the vegetative cell which produces and releases the toxin. The spores only germinate in the absence of oxygen — germination of clostridia requires anaerobic conditions. Clostridia only cause disease under conditions where germination is possible, e.g. in bottled food, in deep wounds.

Disease Pattern: Four important diseases are attributed to the clostridial organisms —

Cl. botulinum	— Botulism (food poisoning)
Cl. tetani	— Tetanus
Cl. perfringens	
Cl. septicum	— Gas gangrene
Cl. novyi (*oedematiens*)	
Cl. perfringens	— Food poisoning

In each the exotoxin secreted is responsible for the disease. The organism is non-invasive except in gas gangrene where limited invasiveness is displayed.

Treatment: Definitive treatment in diseases caused by the secretion of exotoxin may be by the administration of antitoxin. Antitoxin consists of specific antibody, produced occasionally in man but more frequently in animals, against the exotoxin. Administration of these antibodies leads to neutralization of the toxin provided the toxin has not become attached to cells. Once toxin has become attached to cells the antitoxin has no effect and the toxin continues to exert its deleterious effects. If antitoxin is to be administered it must be given early.

Prevention: Depending on the number of toxins produced and the number of antigenic types of toxin, prophylaxis may be possible by immunization using a specific toxoid. Toxoid is a biologically inactive but antigenically unchanged toxin.

Laboratory Diagnosis: The gram stain is of value in identifying Gram-positive bacilli. Spores may also often be seen. Species differentiation is, however, more difficult, e.g. both *Cl. tetani* (pathogen) and *Cl. tetanomorphum* (saphrophyte) have terminal bulging spores and are classically referred to as having a tennis racket shape. The definitive laboratory identification of Gram-positive bacili often involves the use of —

(*a*)   immunological techniques, e.g. the diagnosis of clostridia causing gas gangrene by neutralization tests

(*b*)   laboratory animals, e.g. in the identification of botulism or tetanus.

Clostridium botulinum
(Clostridial food poisoning.)

Source: Spores of *Cl. botulinum* are widely distributed in soil and may contaminate fruit, vegetables, fish and other food products.

Spread: The spores are highly resistant to heat, withstanding temperatures of over 100°C for three hours or more. Adequate cooking of contaminated food will kill all the vegetative forms but will not destroy the clostridial spores. Bottling introduces an anaerobic environment and the spores are given the opportunity to germinate. The vegetative bacteria so produced multiply and produce toxin. The toxin is heat labile and can be destroyed if exposed to 100°C for 10 minutes. Often bottled, canned and vacuum packed foods are eaten without heating.

Virulence: Botulism is due to toxin production. Botulinum toxin is one of the most potent biological toxins known to man — 1μgm or less may kill an adult man. Different types of toxin A-E are recognised. Types A and B are predominantly associated with canned or bottled foods, type E with fish.

Disease Pattern: Botulism is an intoxication. The toxin, if ingested, is absorbed through the mucous membrane of the gastro-intestinal tract. The toxin is not inactivated by the proteolytic enzymes of the gastro-intestinal tract — in fact it may be activated by these enzymes. It may also be absorbed directly through the skin. The toxin once absorbed is thought to attach to the gangliosides of the presynaptic membrane of cholenergic nerves. The toxin-glycoside complex so formed is thought to block the release of acetyl choline — the neurotransmitter. Clinically, paralysis supervenes in 18-24 hours after ingestion of the toxin. Only type E causes nausea and vomiting.

Prevention and Control: Food contaminated by *Cl. botulinum* may appear perfectly good, alternately food that appears "off" need not be contaminated by *Clostridium botulinum*. Although a blown can is not diagnostic of botulism, it may be infected. All blown cans should therefore be discarded as a safety precaution. The canning industry is aware of the dangers of botulism and uses high temperatures (120°C) in the preparation of their products. Nitrates used to preserve meats inhibit the growth of *Cl. botulinum*. (Nitrates converted to nitrites and nitrosamines bear a postulated aetiological association with gastric cancer.) The main danger of botulism today lies in home preserves. These should be boiled for at least 15 minutes immediately prior to use.

Botulism is fatal in over 30% of cases. In each case type specific anti-toxin, if given early enough, could be life saving.

Clostridium tetani

Source: The organism is found in soil and may also be found occasionally in the gastro-intestinal tract of man.

Spread: The organism is spread in the spore form. If introduced into puncture wounds the spore form can germinate and toxin production can start. The spore germinates under anaerobic conditions — deep penetrating wounds, especially those containing foreign material, e.g. soil or bacteria, are especially conducive to the germination of *Cl. tetani*.

Virulence: *Cl. tetani* produces a potent exotoxin, tetanospasmin.

Disease Pattern: Tetanospasmin spreads by the blood stream, plus possibly along nerve axons, to the anterior horn cells of the spinal cord. Spasms and convulsions result.

The spores may remain dormant for long periods and the patient may only present with overt tetanus long after the wound (e.g. caused by a rose thorn) has been forgotten. This condition is termed occult tetanus.

Tetanospasmin differs from botulinum toxin in that:
  (i) Tetanospasmin has only one antigenic type — a single toxoid is therefore protective.
  (ii) It is more heat sensitive — tetanus toxin is inactivated at 65°C for 5 minutes; it is inactivated by proteolytic enzymes.
  (iii) Tetanus is an infection; botulism an intoxication.
  (iv) Tetanus leads to convulsions; botulism to paralysis.

Prevention and Control: *Cl. tetani* are wide spread. Prevention against tetanus is possible by immunization. Protective antibodies are produced against the toxoid. The antibodies neutralize the toxin in the event of infection. Once an individual has had tetanus he still requires a course of immunization. The quantity of the toxin released in natural infection is insufficient to adequately prime the immune system.

Tetanus Neonatorum — this occurs in infants in areas where tribal customs require treatment of the umbilical cord with cowdung. Infection of the cord with *Clostridium tetani* leads to tetanus in the infant. Prophylaxis is best achieved by immunization of the mother. A booster should be given during pregnancy so that the high level of maternal antibodies can filter across the placenta and protect the baby. Health education should be practised but not relied upon in this situation.

Lockjaw is the layman's term for localized tetanus of the jaw.

Clostridium perfringens — gastroenteritis.

Source: *Cl. perfringens* may be found in soil, faeces and contaminated foods, e.g. meat.

Spread: The spores survive normal cooking and germinate as the temperature drops. In the centre of, for example, a piece of meat, anaerobic conditions prevail and allow the spores to germinate. The organism multiples prolifically. Long slow cooling plus storage in warm areas allow sufficient multiplication of the organism to cause disease. A large number of organisms must be ingested before gastroenteritis develops. Cooked meat and poultry are the prime vehicles for the spread of *Cl. perfringens* gastroenteritis.

Virulence: *Clostridium perfringens* produces an enterotoxin when the organism sporulates in the gastro-intestinal tract of the host. Lecithinases are also produced — these are postulated to lead to the production of irritant products. *Cl. perfringens* does not cause an intoxication, it causes an infection. It therefore does not cause true food poisoning but gastroenteritis.

Disease Pattern: After an incubation period of 18 hours the organism, if ingested in sufficient quantities, will have produced sufficient toxin to cause the host to develop profuse diarrhoea.

The Gas Gangrene Clostridia

A number of different species of clostridia are capable of causing gas gangrene. Of those capable of causing gas gangrene *Clostridium perfringes* is the most commonly encountered culprit.

Source: These clostridia are frequently encountered in the intestinal tract of man. Nine out of every ten men excrete clostridial spores in their faeces.

Spread: Like tetanus, the spore once introduced into a wound requires anaerobic conditions for germination. People at risk of developing gas gangrene are —

(i) those with extensive contaminated raw areas, e.g. motor vehicle accidents, war wounds, septic abortions;

(ii) those with vascular disease, e.g. mesenteric thrombosis leading to gas gangrene of the intestine, peripheral vascular disease with contamination of the amputation stump by faecal clostridia. The diabetic is particularly at risk. Infection by these clostridia is often endogenous.

Virulence: The clostridia of gas gangrene secrete a variety of enzymes and toxins. These enzymes and toxins lead to tissue death and necrosis. Death of adjacent tissue facilitates further spread. The clostridia responsible for gas gangrene are the following —

Cl. perfringens, Cl. novyi and *Cl. septicum*

Disease Pattern: There are three forms of clostridial infection — clostridial wound contamination, clostridial cellulitis and clostridial myositis. Clostridial wound contamination is common — more than 80% of wounds are contaminated by clostridia. Provided the wound is superficial and contains no necrotic or foreign material, this presents no problem. The second stage is that of anaerobic cellulitis where a superficial infection with clostridia has occurred. This should be treated but is not life threatening. Clostridial myositis, the last of the trio, is better known as gas gangrene. As the toxins produced by the organism destroy the adjacent muscle cells, spread into these anaerobic areas occurs. Clostridial metabolism leads to the production of gas, e.g. CO_2 and H_2. This is released into the tissues and is responsible for the crepitations felt on palpation. Other organisms, e.g. *E. coli*, klebsiella, bacteroides and peptostreptococci also produce gas and must not be confused with clostridia.

Prevention and Treatment: Prevention of gas gangrene involves removal of clostridia. This can be achieved by adequate debridement of the wound. Hyperbaric oxygen is now being successfully used in the treatment of gas gangrene. Oxygen is toxic to the organism and also prevents germination of spores. Adjuncts to therapy are antibiotics and polyvalent antitoxin. Amputation is all too frequently the last resort used in an attempt to save the patient's life.

Non-sporing Gram-positive bacilli
Propionibacteria

These organisms are skin commensals. *Propionibacterium acnes* may have a role in acne. They are postulated to release lipases which convert skin lipids to free fatty acids. These free fatty acids may cause tissue irritation resulting in inflammation and acne.

Corynebacteria

Corynebacteria are aerobic non-sporing Gram-positive bacilli. They form a group of organisms which includes saphrophytes and pathogens. The saphrophytes, collectively called "diphtheroids", are commensals of respiratory mucosa and conjunctiva. They must be distinguished from the pathogen *C. diphtheriae*.

Corynebacterium diphtheriae

Source: *Corynebacterium diphtheriae* occurs in the respiratory tract and skin of both patients and carriers.

Spread: This is by direct contact, or by droplet infection. The portal of entry could be the throat, nasal mucosa, larynx or rarely a skin wound.

Virulence: The organism multiplies producing a toxin. The toxin induces local epithelial cell death and a superficial inflammatory reaction results. These combine to give the classical clinical picture of a pseudomembrane. The organism does not invade.

Not all *C. diphtheriae* organisms are capable of producing toxin. As diphtheria is a disease caused by a toxin it is important to know whether the organism is toxigenic or not. The ability of the organism to produce toxin depends on:

(i) Infection of the organism by a specific β phage. This is a bacteriophage (viral) infection of a bacterium.

(ii) A low iron content in the bacterial cell facilitates toxin production.

A diphtheria organism which has not been infected by the β phage is harmless until such time as it becomes infected. Once lysogeny by the β phage has occurred the diphtheria organism becomes potentially lethal.

Disease Pattern: The pseudomembrane of diphtheria may be found in the nose, covering the larynx or in the throat. The throat is the most common site. Depending on the site of the membrane the child may complain of a nasal discharge, or a sore throat or may even die of asphyxia. The organism produces toxin as it multiplies. Locally, toxin causes production of the pseudomembrane, absorbed toxin causes the more serious manifestations of diphtheria. The absorbed toxin attaches to cells, notably those of the adrenal, the nervous system and the kidney. Diphtheria toxin has two fractions — fragment B which attaches to the cytoplasmic membrane, and fragment A which diffuses into the cell's cytoplasm. Fragment A acts on the machinery involved in protein synthesis at the level of the ribosomes. It interferes with protein synthesis by preventing elongation of the polypeptide chain.

Prevention and Control: It is public health practice to immunize the population against diphtheria. An individual who has been immunized and is exposed to a toxigenic strain of *C. diphtheriae* may become a carrier but he will not develop clinical disease. He will, however, pose a threat to any individual in the community who has not been protected against diphtheria. Patients who have recovered from diphtheria are therefore subjected to repeated throat swabs. Ideally three consecutive negative throat swabs are required at 24-48 hour intervals prior to discharge of a diphtheria case.

Control of diphtheria in a community is based on immunization and on the control of carriers. Swabbing diphtheria contacts and Schick testing of high risk individuals and contacts is routinely performed in certain areas.

Treatment: The early administration of antitoxin is essential. The diagnosis of diphtheria is thus a clinical one. The laboratory can confirm the clinical diagnosis. The antibiotic of choice is penicillin.

Laboratory Findings: The laboratory used a special stain when trying to morphologically identify a member of the genus Corynebacterium. Both Ponders' stain and Albert's stain are of value. *Corynebacteria diphtheriae* have metachromatic granules and classically lie in the form of chinese letters. Differentiation of this organism from the diphtheroids is based on their sugar reactions. Once the organism has been identified as *C. diphtheriae* it is necessary to perform immunodiffusion tests to show whether the strain isolated produces toxin or not.

Certain characteristics shared by Gram-positive bacilli

(1) Penicillin is the antibiotic of choice.

(2) Exotoxin production is a major mechanism of disease induction.

(3) Specific therapy must be instituted early.

Once the exotoxin has attached to its target cell, no therapy is available to reverse its action. Neutralization of the effects of exotoxin must be achieved prior to the attachment of the toxin to the cell.

It is therefore contra-indicated to wait for laboratory confirmation of a clinical diagnosis of tetanus, gas gangrene or diphtheria. Specific therapy is an attempt to neutralize the toxin with specific antitoxin. A complication attributable to the use of horse antiserum (antitoxin) is serum sickness. The incidence of severe side effects increases with subsequent exposures to horse serum. It is therefore necessary to ensure that any individual who has had horse serum once, be protected as far as possible, from requiring horse serum a second time. This is achieved by immunizing the patient against diphtheria and tetanus. Repeated intra-venous exposure to foreign protein can be fatal.

The extent of the clinical disease will determine the use of antibiotics and supportive therapy.

(4) The disease produced by secretion of a specific exotoxin is often characteristic of the organism producing the toxin, i.e. the disease is organism specific.

(5) Exotoxins are potent toxins. Public health measures may be employed to control the spread of organisms capable of secreting these toxins.

(6) Control of these diseases is often based on immunization. Immunization is based on exposure of the individual's immune system to a specific toxoid. The treated toxin or toxoid is harmless. The toxoid primes the individual's immune system which is then enabled to recognise the toxin and react protectively on future exposure. An immunization programme involves repeated exposure to the toxoid during primary immunization in order to speed up and improve both the quantitative and the qualitative immune response of the host. Routine immunization against tetanus and diphtheria is practised in many countries. Individuals exposed to an occupational risk of anthrax or botulism are immunized against these diseases.

GRAM-NEGATIVE BACILLI

All Gram-negative bacilli have lipopolysaccharide in their cell walls. The polysaccharide portion is antigenic, the lipid portion, termed Lipid A, is toxic. Endotoxic shock is associated with Gram-negative septicaemia. The organisms lyse in the blood stream and release their lipopolysaccharide (endotoxin).

Endotoxin has the following effects:
  (i) It causes the release of endogenous pyrogens from members of the white cell series. The result is pyrexia.

(ii) The combined effects of endotoxin and infection lead to changes in the leucocyte count.

(iii) Release of kinins, histamine, serotonin and the activation of complement contribute to an imbalance between the blood volume and the vasculature capacity. This results in a drop in blood pressure.

(iv) Endotoxin activates both blood coagulation and fibrinolysis (clot lysis). This may lead to disseminated intravascular coagulation with haemorrhage.

(v) Irreversible shock may lead to the death of the patient.

The response of the individual to endotoxin may be modified by his immune response. Many Gram-negative bacilli are normal inhabitants of man's intestinal tract. Man's exposure to the lipopolysaccharide in his intestine may exaggerate his response on subsequent exposure to endotoxin in his blood stream.

Salmonella

There are two important groups of salmonellae — those which cause typhoid fever and those which cause gastroenteritis. The salmonellae causing typhoid in man are human pathogens, those causing gastroenteritis in man are animal pathogens.

Salmonella typhi

Source: Man is the animal that contaminates water and food supplies with *Salmonella typhi*. Both patients and carriers excrete the typhoid organism in their faeces or urine. Faecal shedders are ten times more important as culprits in the spread of *Salmonella typhi* than are carriers excreting the organism in their urine.

Spread: *Salmonella typhi* can be spread by food but is more usually spread by water. Water borne typhoid is usually as a result of contamination of the water supply by man.

Virulence: *Salmonella typhi* and hence typhoid are world wide. The organism only causes disease in man. The organism is resistant to digestion by macrophages. It resides in the macrophage which protects it against the host's circulating antibody and also makes it difficult for antimicrobial agents to reach the organism. *S. typhi* has endotoxin within its cell wall.

Disease Pattern: After man has ingested the contaminated water or food the organism passes into the intestine and invades the bowel wall. The infective dose of *S. typhi* is 100 000 organisms. During the 7-14 day incubation period the organisms penetrate the bowel wall and spread by the blood stream to the liver, spleen and other reticulo-endothelial tissue. Clinical symptoms coincide with the second bacteraemic phase when the organism reaches the skin, the central nervous system and the gastro-intestinal tract. The skin rash — rose spots, the headache, and the bloated constipated feeling associated with typhoid occur at this stage.

Depending on the stage of the disease the organism may be isolated from one or more of the following sites — blood, stool and/or urine. Serological tests, for antibodies against the organism, become positive during the second week of illness. The typhoid patient develops high levels of antibodies against the organism but the organism lies protected inside macrophages.

Treatment: Typhoid may be treated with ampicillin, co-trimoxazole or chloramphenicol. In view of the mortality associated with typhoid, e.g. due to haemorrhage, perforation or shock, the use of chloramphenicol is justified in spite of the hazard of bone marrow depression.

Prevention and Control: Typhoid is not a contagious disease. It is not spread directly from person to person. It requires a period in either water or food in order to multiply and reach an adequate number to constitute an infective dose. In areas of poor hygiene, typhoid outbreaks are usually water borne; food borne typhoid is associated with better socio-economic conditions.

Adequate sanitation, regular water analysis for faecal contamination and follow-up of both cases and carriers are important principles in typhoid control. Routine checks on food handlers are also carried out. Typhoid carriers discovered amongst food handlers must not be permitted to continue working with food until they are declared free of the organism.

Vaccination is also practised against typhoid but is not entirely effective.

Typhoid or enteric fever is caused not only by *Salmonella typhi* but to a lesser extent by *Salmonella paratyphi* A and B.

Salmonella gastroenteritis

Source: Salmonella producing gastroenteritis in man are primary animal pathogens. They may be transmitted from animals to man in animal products, e.g. meat, eggs, etc. There are a multitude of different salmonella capable of causing gastroenteritis in man — many are named according to the geographical area in which they were first identified, e.g. *Salmonella johannesburg, Salmonella london*. As a group the organisms responsible for gastroenteritis are referred to as *Salmonella species*.

Spread: The organisms are frequently ingested in pork, less frequently in beef. Processed meat is a greater hazard than fresh meat. Raw milk is a danger — it can act as a vehicle of spread not only of brucellosis and tuberculosis but also of salmonella gastroenteritis. Egg products — particularly custards, cakes and egg nogs — can lead to outbreaks of salmonellosis. Salmonella gastroenteritis has occurred in hospitals due to the preparation of egg nogs with contaminated eggs.

Virulence: The organisms are less well adapted to man than *Salmonella typhi*. Their infective dose is 10^9 organisms. The organisms illicit an inflammation response in the lamina propria of the terminal ileum.

Disease Pattern: Symptoms develop 8-24 hours after ingestion of contaminated food and constitutional symptoms are prominent. The patient complains of headache and fever. Diarrhoea may be mild or fulminant. Unlike food poisoning caused by staphylococci, nausea and vomiting are not prominant.

Treatment: This is supportive. Fluids and electrolyte solutions should replace those lost. Antibiotics are not indicated as they prolong the carrier state.

Prevention and Control: Prevention of salmonellosis starts at the level of animal husbandry. Animals transported to the abbatoir should be subject to minimal stress.

Spread of salmonellae is exaggerated if fearful animals are cooped up in trucks. The separation of the gastrointestinal tract and its contents from muscles and other organs during slaughter is important. The housewife and foodhandler can minimize the opportunity for multiplication of any organism which has contaminated the food by deep freezing and adequate thawing prior to use. Adequate cooking is a simple way of killing these organisms and preventing disease.

Shigella

Source: These Gram-negative bacilli are spread from patients by direct contact or by flies, fomites and food.

Spread: An individual suffering from bacillary dysentry after passing a dysenteric stool may contaminate his hands, the doorknob and the tap before washing his hands. A healthy individual may handle the tap and suck his now contaminated finger. The infective dose of shigella is 10 000 organisms. They do not require a period of multiplication before infecting a new host. They are susceptible to drying and heat but will survive for many weeks on moist toilet seats.

Virulence: Shigella are postulated to cause disease by their ability to invade the superficial epithelial cells and also by their ability to cause the release of prostaglandins from the cells of the small intestine. Prostaglandins are thought to stimulate adenyl cyclase, an enzyme which stimulates the release of fluid and electrolytes into the lumen of the small bowel.

Disease Pattern: The clinical picture will be determined by the strain of shigella involved and also by the area of bowel involved. There are four strains of shigella responsible for bacillary dysentery in man. These are *Shigella dysenteriae, Shigella sonnei, Shigella flexneri* and *Shigella boydii*. If the predominant lesion is in the small intestine the dysentry will simulate diarrhoea; if the predominant lesion is in the large bowel a frank dysentry will result. Dysentry differs from diarrhoea in that blood, mucus and cells are present in the stool.

Treatment: Antibiotic therapy is not contra-indicated as is the case in salmonellosis.

Prevention and Control: Control of shigellosis or bacillary dysentry is at the level of personal hygiene. In adults outbreaks are usually self limiting. Children often require treatment.

Vibrio

There are two vibrios of importance to man. *V. cholerae*, the organism responsible for cholera, that devastating disease with the rice water stool, and *V. parahaemolyticus*, an organism causing gastroenteritis.

Vibrio cholerae

Source: Man is the source of *V. cholerae*. Carriers contaminate water supplies.

Spread: Cholera is usually spread by water. Occasionally in certain arid regions cholera has been shown to be spread by direct contact.

Virulence: Both the classical and El tor biotypes give rise to fulminating diarrhoea. The organism in both cases is non-invasive and causes disease by secretion of enterotoxin.

Disease Pattern: Ingestion by a healthy person of 10^8 or 10^9 organisms leads to clinically overt disease. The organisms are sensitive to acid and many demise in the stomach. Those which survive and reach the small intestine multiply in the lumen of the intestine. Adherence to the epithelial cells of the small intestine is required before the organisms can start to secrete their enterotoxin. Enterotoxin, an exotoxin, stimulates the production of adenyl cyclase which in turn leads to the secretion of fluid and electrolytes into the bowel lumen. Absorption, which remains normal, is masked by the excess out-pouring of fluid. Enterotoxin is therefore responsible for a fulmi-nating diarrhoea. Patients dying of cholera do so due to an exces-sive loss of fluid and electrolytes.

Management: Dehydration and shock must be prevented. This is achieved by the restoration of fluids and electrolytes by either the oral or intravenous routes. Special "metabolic beds" with a cavity in the buttock region are available. The watery stool flows directly from the patient into a calibrated bucket. Exact fluid loss is noted and the patient is not persistently disturbed. The collecting bucket should contain a known volume of disinfectant to destroy the bacilli excreted in the stool.

Tetracyclines may be used to eradicate the organisms present in the patient's bowel.

Prevention and Control: Cholera is often quoted as the disease best demonstrating the iceberg phenomenon. For every one clinical case of cholera there are nine sub-clinical infections.

Health education and the correct handling of sewage is necessary in cholera endemic areas. *V. cholerae* can survive for 24 hours in sewage; it is sensitive to disinfectants, including chlorine.

Cholera immunization is no longer required by International Health Authorities for travellers. This ruling is based on the observation that the value of immunization is limited — it is of limited value to the individual and of no value to the general public. Immunization against cholera will prevent some individuals who come in contact with the organism from developing the disease, but it will not stop them from becoming carriers and spreading the organism. The taking of prophylactic antibiotics by travellers is frowned upon as this leads to alteration of the normal microbial flora in the intestinal tract and also selects for antibiotic resistant strains of bacteria.

Cholera control depends on good sanitation, an adequate surveillance in cholera receptive areas and on the early diagnosis of cases and carriers. Early diagnosis and adequate treatment can reduce the mortality rate to zero. Early identification of carriers and constant checks on water supplies can prevent epidemics.

Vibrio parahaemolyticus

Source: This organism is found in the sea and contaminates sea food. In Japan *V. parahaemolyticus* is responsible for 80% of infective gastroenteritis. In other countries microbiologists seldom incriminate this organism as a contaminant of food. This is probably not because the organisms are not present but rather because it is missed on routine testing. The organisms require a selective culture medium with a high salt content.

Spread: The organism is spread by the ingestion of fresh sea food.

Virulence: The pathogenesis of the organism has not been well worked out. Enterotoxin is not thought to play a role.

Disease Pattern: Gastroenteritis develops 12-15 hours after the ingestion of fish. The patient usually has diarrhoea but may occasionally pass a blood stained stool. *V. parahaemolyticus* causes an infection, not an intoxication.

Treatment: The illness is usually self limiting, recovery occurring in one to two days.

Escherichia

Escherichia coli

Source: *E. coli* is a normal inhabitant of the bowel.

Spread: *E. coli* may cause disease by being removed from its normal anatomical site and being introduced into a normally sterile area, e.g. meningies, bladder, blood. In these cases *E. coli* is behaving as an opportunistic pathogen. *E. coli* can under certain circumstances behave as a true pathogen and cause disease in its normal anatomical site. These *E. coli* strains are not commensals of that individual's bowel and are possibly derived from an infected water source.

Virulence: Certain strains of *E. coli* are capable of causing disease by secretion of an enterotoxin. These strains are infected by an extraneous piece of nuclear material termed a plasmid. The plasmid confers the ability to produce enterotoxin on the infected bacterium. Another strain of *E. coli* is capable of invading the superficial cells lining the gastro-intestinal tract. All *E.coli* are Gram-negative and therefore capable of releasing endotoxin on lysis.

Disease Pattern: Certain strains of *E. coli* are capable of producing diarrhoea — diarrhoea in infants is thought to often be due to enteropathogenic *E. coli*. Invasive *E. coli* can cause a dysentry-like picture. Any strain of *E. coli* introduced into a normally sterile site can cause opportunistic infection, e.g. urinary tract infection, neonatal meningitis, septicaemia.

E. coli and water — *E. coli* constitute a group of organisms regularly found in faeces. The presence of *E. coli* in a river, dam or stream is therefore an index of faecal contamination of that water. Tests are regularly performed to detect the presence of *E. coli* in water used for human consumption. Water containing *E. coli* is condemned, not because of this organism *per se* but because faecal contamination of the water has occurred. The faecally polluted water is suspect — it may be a source of cholera or typhoid.

OPPORTUNISTIC GRAM-NEGATIVE BACILLI

A large number of Gram-negative bacilli are capable of causing disease in hosts with an impaired resistance. This impaired resistance may be:

(i) At the level of a superficial barrier, e.g. in burns the organism bypasses the skin barrier; organism may be introduced into the bladder on a contaminated catheter or by trauma of the urethra.

(ii) It may be related to defects in non-specific immunity, e.g. a congenital defect of leucocytes, a rubeola induced defect in polymorph chemotaxis.

(iii) It may be at the level of specific immunity, e.g. Hodgkin's disease, cancer, iatrogenic depression of immunity due to steroid therapy.

Only three members of these Gram-negative organisms classified as potential pathogens are to be discussed. All these organisms can present problems in the hospital environment. The three groups to be discussed are:

Klebsiella
Proteus
Pseudomonas

Klebsiella

Source: Klebsiella are found in the environment. They are normally found in soil and must be differentiated in water testing so as to avoid misidentification as *E. coli*.

Virulence: These organisms resist phagocytosis due to the presence of a large capsule.

Disease Pattern: *Klebsiella pneumoniae* is the most pathogenic of the species and may act as a primary invader causing Klebsiella or Friedlander's pneumonia. This may be fatal. Diabetic and alcoholic patients are particularly at risk.

Infections with klebsiella organisms are on the increase in the hospital situation. This increase runs hand in hand with the increase in immuno-suppression used in transplantation and the increase of cancer chemotherapy. The persistent and often indiscriminate use of antibiotics exaggerates the problem of nosocomial klebsiella infections.

Klebsiella organisms can act as opportunistic invaders in urinary tract infections in bronchopneumonia, in osteomyelitis, etc.

Other members of the *Enterobacteriaceae* family (serratia and enterobacter) are also increasingly listed as hospital acquired infections. They are more resistant than klebsiella to antibiotic therapy.

Proteus

There are four species in this group. All are motile but two are so actively motile that if grown on one side of a solid medium they will spread over the whole surface of the medium. This is termed swarming.

Source: Proteus organisms are widespread in the environment. They are found in soil and in sewage.

Disease Pattern: One member of this group of opportunists is suspected, but not proven, of causing diarrhoea. All the members of this group are well recognised as urinary tract pathogens. Once these opportunists have gained entrance to the bladder they split urea and make the urine alkali. The ammonia so produced may inactivate complement, thus compromising the host's defences.

Urinary tract infections due to proteus are common in both the hospital and the community. Proteus bacteraemia and wound sepsis are a hospital problem.

Pseudomonas

Source: The green film found in many hospital and household drains may be nothing less than a pseudomonas culture. Pseudomonas species has included amongst its members an organism, *Pseudomonas aeruginosa*, which is easily recognised by its green pigment. Pseudomonas is an organism found in water. It proliferates freely in drains and sinks.

Disease Pattern: Pseudomonas prefers hosts with some defect in their immune system. The immunosuppressed host provides the organism with a new play-ground. It frequently causes systemic disease in these patients. Localized infections, e.g. of the eye due to the use of contaminated eyedrops, or of bedsores due to washing with utensils from contaminated sinks, do occur.

The patient with burns is at particular risk — local infection followed by septicaemia and death is a sadly familiar sequence. In the paraplegic patient pseudomonas is a formidible cause of urinary tract infection.

Pseudomonas does not exclusively cause infection in hospitals. It does, however, produce about 200 hospital infections to every one community infection. Pseudomonas, an organism which multiplies in damp areas, is a most important cause of nosocomial infections.

THE SMALL GRAM-NEGATIVE BACILLI

The small Gram-negative bacilli have been grouped together as *Parvobacteriaceae* or *Brucellaceae*. Among this group of bacteroides, an anaerobic organism which is the predominant bacterium of the normal intestinal flora. Of the group of small Gram-negative organisms only four members will be considered:

Haemophilus ⎱	These organisms have specific cultural require-
Bordetella ⎰	ments.
Brucella ⎫	These organisms usually cause disease in animals but
⎬	may be transmitted to man, i.e. they may be classi-
Yersinia ⎭	fied as zoonoses.

Haemophilus

These are pleomorphic Gram-negative coccobacilli. They depend on one or two factors for their normal growth. The X factor (haemin, found in red blood cells) and the V factor (a coenzyme NAD or NADP) are necessary for normal metabolism. The V factor can be produced by certain organisms amongst which are staphylococci. Identification of *Haemophilus influenzae* can be definitely made by culturing the organism on a blood agar plate and seeing if the colonies are larger and more numerous in the vicinity of a staphylococcal streak culture. This phenomenon is termed satellitism.

Figure 20
SATELLITISM

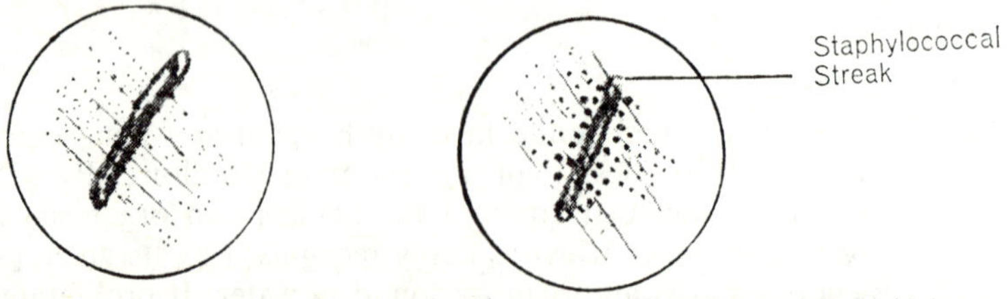

E. *coli* does not show satellitism

H. *influenzae* showing satellitism

Staphylococcal Streak

Haemophilus aegypticus, also called Koch-Weeks bacillus, is an important cause of conjunctivitis. This form of conjunctivitis is highly communicable, especially amongst small children.

Haemophilus ducreyi is spread venereally. It is the causative organism of chancroid or soft sore. Chancroid presents as an ulcer on the genitalia and has associated tender draining lymph nodes. Treatment for this venereal disease is sulphonamides.

Haemophilus influenzae

Source and spread: Varieties of non-encapsulated *H. influenzae* are found in the throat and nasopharynx of 60-80% of children. Spread of *H. influenzae* is person-to-person by droplets. The patient with haemophilus meningitis is a far less important source of infection than the carrier.

Virulence: These organisms only cause disease in the face of a decreased host resistance. The types of *H. influenzae* causing severe disease are encapsulated. Their capsules protect them against phagocytosis.

Disease Pattern: *H. influenzae* is an important pathogen in children. It is the commonest cause of acute bacterial meningitis in early childhood. Late neurological and intellectual impairment following influenzal meningitis are well recognised. The peak incidence occurs between 2 months and 3 years of age. *H. influenzae* can cause fatal acute epiglottitis in the 2 to 7 year age group. Acute oedema of the epiglottis can block the respiratory passages resulting in asphyxia. Tracheostomy may be life saving.

In the adult, *H. influenzae* is thought to play a role in exacerbacians of chronic bronchitis.

Haemophilus influenzae and *Streptococcus pneumoniae* have certain similar characteristics.
   (i) There are high carrier rates in the upper respiratory tract of the relatively non-pathogenic forms, while there is a low carrier rate of the virulent variety.
  (ii) Immunity depends on the production of antibodies to capsular antigen.
 (iii) Their pathogenicity depends on their ability to resist phagocytosis. This ability is related to the presence of their capsules. There is antigenic cross-reactivity of the capsular polysaccharide amongst certain types of *H. influenzae* and pneumococci.
 (iv) Diseases caused by these organisms may involve either the respiratory system or the meningis.
  (v) Both are spread by droplet infection.
 (vi) Both groups contain members which are primary pathogens and virulent; other members are opportunists.

Bordetella

Source and Spread: Bordetella is an organism causing disease in man. It is spread from man to man by droplets. These organisms are very fastidious — special collection and culture techniques are necessary if the organism is to be isolated.

Virulence: During the incubation period of 1-2 weeks the organism multiplies. It does not cause disease by invasion but by the secretion of toxins.

Disease Pattern: *Bordetella pertussis* and *Bordetella parapertussis* are responsible for respiratory infection during childhood. *Bordetella pertussis* is responsible for the more severe disease. The clinical picture of bordetella infection is characterized by a paroxysm of coughing followed by a long inspiration. The disease is called whooping cough. All that whoops is not whooping cough — certain viruses, e.g. the adenovirus, can give a similar picture.

Whooping cough is characterized by three phases:
the catarrhal phase
the whooping or paroxysmal phase
the convalescent phase.

Each phase lasts about two weeks. The patient is infectious during the first two to three weeks. During the whooping phase bronchioli can be blocked by mucus plugs and areas of atalectasis can occur. Collapsed areas of lung are susceptible to secondary infection. If sufficient atalectasis occurs, hypoxia can become a problem. Vomiting and convulsions are a feature of whooping cough.

Treatment: Antibiotics, unless administered during the incubation period, do not alter the course of the pertussis infection. Penicillin is, however, usually given to whooping cough patients — this will have no effect on bordetella, it is administered as prophylaxis against secondary infection. Deaths associated with whooping cough are usually attributed to secondary infection.

Prevention and Control: The mother is incapable of transplacentally transferring protective antibody against whooping cough. Infants less than 6 months of age are therefore particularly at risk. Immunization against whooping cough is usually started when the infant is 3 months of age. The triple vaccine against whooping cough, tetanus and diphtheria is routinely given to infants. Whooping cough vaccine is not 100 per cent protective.

Brucella

There are a number of brucella species — the most important pathogen in man is *Brucella melitensis*.

Source: Brucella is a disease of animals which can be spread to man. The species of brucella is determined by the animal infected, e.g. *Brucella suis* infects pigs, *Brucella melitensis* sheep and goats, *Brucella abortus* cattle and *Brucella canis* dogs.

Spread: Brucella is spread by direct contact with abraded epidermal areas and mucous membranes including the conjunctiva. Aerosol spread is suspected.

Virulence: The organism is resistant to digestion by phagocytes. It is an intracellular pathogen.

Disease Pattern: Brucellosis is a diagnostic challenge. The onset is insidious and the presentation often that of a pyrexia of unknown origin. Chronic cases of brucellosis are often mis-diagnosed as psychiatric problems. Arthritis is a feature of the disease.

Prevention and Control: As brucellosis can often be acquired from unpasteurized milk or infected animal carcasses, vets, farmers and abattoir workers are the population at risk. Immunization for at risk workers is available, but the vaccine has side effects. Control of herds can be achieved by immunization of the herds with a live attenuated vaccine. Milk should be pasteurized. In certain countries brucellosis is a notifiable disease.

Yersinia

Yersinia pestis

Yersinia pestis is a small Gram-negative bacillus which exhibits bipolar staining. It is the causative organism of plague. Plague is a zoonosis.

Spread: *Yersinia pestis* is spread to man in one of two ways:
  (*a*) The bite of a flea inoculating the bacillus.
  (*b*) More rarely, and only during epidemics, by droplet inhalation from a human with pneumonic plague.

Virulence: The infective dose of *Yersinia pestis* is one. *Yersinia pestis* has some ability to resist phagocytosis. It secretes a variety of virulence factors. Pesticin and fraction 1 (only produced at 37°C) provide a lethal combination.

Disease Pattern: Man rarely, if ever, recovers from pneumonic or septicaemic plague. He may, however, resist death in the case of bubonic plague. Should the local nymph node fail to localize the infection, blood spread will rapidly convert bubonic plague into the more sinister septicaemic plague.

In any isolated population, bubonic plague precedes pneumonic plague. Failure to localize the organism in the draining lymph node leads to systemic spread. Infection of the lungs is followed by respiratory spread of the organism. The organism spread by the flea is less virulent than the organism spread by droplet infection. The organism spread from man to man has fraction 1 as one of its virulent factors.

Treatment: Tetracyclines are used in the treatment of plague. The early
diagnosis and treatment of plague can be life-saving.

Prevention and Control: Plague outbreaks can be predicted by observing
the rodent population. When an increase in the rodent population
is followed by a high death rate amongst rodents, then plague should
be suspected. Plague is spread by fleas from the wild rodent population to the semi-domestic rodents, from the semi-domestic rodents
to the domestic rodents, and from the domestic rodents to man.

Figure 21
THE SPREAD OF *YERSINIA PESTIS*
FROM WILD RODENTS TO MAN

Wild rodent — (gerbils) *Tatera brandsii*
↓
flea
↓
Semi-domestic rodents (multimammate mouse) *Mastomys natalensis*
↓
flea
↓
Domestic rat — *Rattus rattus*
↓
flea
↓
Man
↓
flea or droplet infection
↓
Man

As each population dies the number becomes depleted so that the fleas,
e.g. *Xenopsylla cheopis* leave their dying host and seek new healthy com-
panions. They carry *Yersinia pestis* from one population to the next
leaving disaster in their wake. *Yersinia pestis* kills rodents, man and also
the fleas.

Man is at risk of exposure to plague if:

(*a*) he goes into the forests and contacts wild rodents;

(*b*) if he is exposed to infected rats and fleas in his home and city.

Control depends on the separation of man from domestic rodents.
Houses and other buildings are ratproofed. Rat poisons and traps are
used on the outskirts of cities to catch rats in order to test them and their
fleas bacteriologically and serologically for the presence of *Yersinia pestis*.
This continual surveillance system gives early warning of a plague epidemic.

Persons who have been in contact with suspected plague are immediately treated with tetracyclines. Suspected plague is treated first and the
diagnosis confirmed later.

Vaccination against plague involves the use of dead organisms.

Yersinia enterocolitica

Man may present with a variety of symptoms, e.g. mesenteric adenitis,
regional ileitis and arthritis.

MYCOBACTERIA

This group of organisms consists of those organisms capable of resisting decolourization by acid and alcohol. This differentiation depends on the of the Ziehl-Neelsen stain.

Three broad groups can be differentiated:

(a) Those which cause tuberculosis —
   M. tuberculosis — human tuberculosis
   M. bovis   — cattle tuberculosis
   M. avium   — bird tuberculosis

(b) Those which cause leprosy —
   M. leprae

(c) A group of atypical mycobacteria (Mott bacilli). This group of organism have pathogens and saphrophytes amongst their members. Pathogens cause diseases of the lung, skin or lymph nodes. They do not cause disease in laboratory animals, e.g. guinea pigs, rabbits.

The atypical mycobacteria have been classed into 2 groups:

(i) The rapid growers — visible colonies are cultured in 4-7 days.

(ii) The slow growers — 3 to 6 weeks are necessary before colonies become visible to the naked eye. These colonies will fall into one of the following groups according to their pigment production:

   (a) The non-chromogenic group — this group fails to produce pigment.

   (b) The scotochromogenic group — this group produces pigment.

   (c) The photochromogenic group — this group only produces pigment if exposed to light.

The mycobacteria form a group of organisms capable of resisting digestion by phagocytes. These organisms survive and multiply in cells of the reticulo-endothelial system. Bacteria which are found surviving inside cells are associated with chronic disease. Extracellular bacteria are usually associated with a more acute type of illness. Specific host defences are adapted to cope differently with different types of infection — cell mediated immunity is more important in intracellular infections, humoral immunity in extracellular infections.

Table XXVII

SPECIFIC IMMUNITY AND THE SITE OF THE ORGANISM

	INTRACELLULAR ORGANISM	EXTRACELLULAR ORGANISM
Specific host defence	Cell mediated immunity	Humoral immunity
Disease	Chronic	Acute

Mycobacterium tuberculosis

World figures show that approximately three million people die of tuberculosis every year. This is a chronic devastating disease.

Spread: *Mycobacterium tuberculosis* is spread by droplet infection.

Disease Pattern: There are two risks associated with the acquisition of tuberculosis. There is the risk associated with exposure to the organism — this risk is especially high in medical personnel coming into contact with undiagnosed tuberculosis. The risk of developing disease is especially high in those groups who have a defect in cell mediated immunity, e.g. those who are on steroids, have leukemia or are malnourished.

As *M. tuberculosis* is usually inhaled, the primary lesion is commonly in lung parenchyma with spread to, and enlargement of, the hilar lymph nodes. *M. bovis* may be spread to man in unpasteurized milk. Ingestion of infected milk leads to infection of the intestine with spread to, and enlargement of, the mesenteric lymph nodes. Tuberculosis is usually held in check by the host's defences — when these fail, generalized spread of the organism can occur, resulting in miliary tuberculosis.

Diagnosis: The diagnosis of tuberculosis is essential from both the public health and personal points of view. An individual with pulmonary tuberculosis spreads the disease. Treatment of the individual rapidly renders him non-infectious. Population surveys to find undiagnosed cases of tuberculosis are carried out. The techniques commonly used are:

(*a*) X-ray screening — this is the least effective means of diagnosis.

(*b*) Skin testing.

(*c*) Sputum testing

Skin Testing: This is based on the interpretation of the host's response to an extract of *M. tuberculosis*. Purified protein derivative (PPD) is an antigenic extract of the human tuberculosis organism. The response to the intradermal inoculation of PPD into the forearm of an individual is recorded 48-72 hours after injection.

If the individual has been previously exposed to, and reacted against, the bacterium, his immune system recognises the antigen and the skin reflects this recognition. The PPD administered stimulates the memory cells of the host's cell mediated immune system and lymphocytes arrive at the site of the foreign antigen in 2-3 days. An area of reddening and induration indicates previous exposure and adequate resistance against the organism. An area of dermal necrosis implies active tuberculosis. False positive and false negative results do occur.

Sputum Testing: The bacteriological method of diagnosis is the most satisfactory. Staining of the sputum with the Ziehl-Neelsen stain may reveal the presence of acid-fast bacilli. To determine whether these acid-fast bacilli are *M. tuberculosis* or not, it is necessary to culture the organism and do biochemical tests. A positive slide indicates many mycobacteria are being shed — positive microscopy requires a concentration of about 10 000 organisms per millilitre of sputum. Once a patient has been diagnosed as having tuberculosis, microscopy is a valuable tool in following the patient's progress.

A provisional identification, i.e. the observation of acid-fast bacilli, becomes available within hours after sending in the specimen. A definitive identification of *M. tuberculosis* takes 6-8 weeks. This delay is due to the slow multiplication of these bacilli.

Immunization: In populations or groups at risk it is advisable to immunize against tuberculosis. Medical personnel in a country where tuberculosis is prevalent should all be skin tested (e.g. the Heaf or Mantoux test). If negative, these individuals should be protected against tuberculosis by immunization.

BCG (Bacillus Calmette Guerin) is the name of the preparation used to immunize against tuberculosis. It consists of a viable, attenuated strain of *M. bovis*. Due to the cross reactivity between *M. tuberculosis* and *M. bovis*, BCG gives some protection against human tuberculosis.

Treatment: Today tuberculosis is a treatable condition. Drug therapy is based on three principles:

(*a*) It must be uninterrupted.

(*b*) Multiple drugs are used simultaneously — three drugs are often combined.

(*c*) Prolonged therapy is essential.

Tuberculosis is treated by continuous, prolonged combined drug therapy.

M. leprae

Leprosy is a chronic disease caused by an organism which has not yet been successfully cultured in artificial media. The organism has been cultivated in the footpads of mice and in the nine banded armadillo.

Source and Spread: *M. tuberculosis* takes 20 hours to multiply, *M. leprae* is thought to take longer. Leprosy is only communicable after prolonged close contact. The nasal mucosa and skin are thought to be the main source of spread.

Disease Pattern: Leprosy is a disease characterized by differences in the host's immune response. On the one hand, if the host lacks an adequate cell mediated immune response the organism multiplies prolifically — this is clinically diagnosed as lepromatous leprosy. These patients are infectious. On the other hand, the host may exhibit an exaggerated immune response to the bacillus. The organisms are rapidly killed. The exaggerated response leads to tissue destruction in the host. The tissues most severely affected are the nerves. Tuberculoid leprosy is characterised by anaesthesia, contractures and deformity. This patient is not infectious.

SPIROCHAETES — THE SPIRAL ORGANISMS

These large spiral organisms may be pathogenic or saphrophytic. The family containing pathogenic members includes those organisms causing syphilis and relapsing fever.

The organisms are coiled and move by twisting without the aid of flagellae. These spiral organisms stain poorly and are therefore usually examined under dark field microscopy or using immunofluorescence. These organisms are difficult to propagate in the laboratory as they require specially enriched media. *Treponema pallidum*, the organism causing syphilis, fails to grow on artificial culture media. The spirochaetes are sensitive to penicillin.

Treponema pallidum

Source: *Treponema pallidum* is an organism adapted to man and spread by man.

Spread: This spirochaete is a delicate organism. It is sensitive to drying and is killed by temperatures of 42°C and over. An organism so sensitive to environmental conditions requires a special mode of transmission. *T. pallidum* is transmitted by direct contact. The organism penetrates intact mucosa or skin abrasions. Syphilis is a venereal disease.

Virulence: *Treponema pallidum* appears to resist phagocytosis but is susceptible to immune lysis. Complement plus specific antibody can react with these organisms and cause their death.

Disease Pattern: Once the organism reaches its new host it multiplies at its site of entry. The multiplication time is relatively long and the incubation period varies between 2-9 weeks. Syphilis presents clinically as a disease with three stages:

Primary syphilis — A local lesion appears at the site of inoculation. This is often described as a punched out ulcer. The primary chancre is painless and infectious. The draining lymph nodes are enlarged, hard and painless. The chancre is often on the genitalia and the nodes in the groin.

Secondary syphilis — here systemic spread of the organism has led to multiple infectious foci, e.g. skin rashes, mucous patches. The nursing staff should handle these patients with gloved hands as tiny abrasions on the attendant's hands can become infected from the syphilitic patient's skin rash.

Tertiary syphilis — this can occur 20 years after the initial infection. Here the host's defences respond to the organism with localized granuloma formation. Cell mediated immunity is expressed destructively and the patient responds to his chronic infection with a delayed hypersensitivity response. The presence of destructive lesions in different anatomical sites can lead to the destruction of various cells, e.g. brain cells, leading to general paralysis of the insane; elastic tissue in the aortic arch, leading to dilatation and rupture of the aorta.

Treponema pallidum can spread across the placenta. Children are born mentally defective, blind and deaf, thanks to a promiscuous parent. Congenital syphilis is a preventable condition if pregnant females are screened, diagnosed and treated early.

Treatment: Penicillin is the drug of choice.

Borrelia

These organisms cause relapsing fever.

Source and Spread: *Borrelia duttoni* is transmitted by the bite of a tick. *Borrelia recurrentis* is transmitted by a body louse. The organisms are released from the louse's coelomic cavity when the host crushes the louse. In so doing the host introduces the organisms into the skin defect created by the louse's bite.

Virulence: The host's defences against relapsing fever are impaired due to two mechanisms employed by the organism —
  (i) The organism breaches the host's superficial defences — the intact skin barrier is breached by the bite of the arthropod.
 (ii) The organism evades the host's specific humoral defences by changing its superficial antigenic structure. The host's defences therefore remain one step behind that of the organism's ingenuity.

    This phenomenon accounts for the relapses classical of this condition.

Disease Pattern: The organism causes fever in man. The attacks of pyrexia may recur up to ten times.

Leptospirosis

Source: These spiral organisms cause disease in animals. Accidental transmission to man may occur — usually by contact with contaminated animal products or excreta.

Spread: The organism is spread from the contaminated source, e.g. a sewer, the dock area where rat urine contaminates the water, by direct contact with abraded or scratched skin.

Disease Pattern: The organism multiplies in the blood causing a leptospiraemia. It is later isolated from urine — leptospiruria.

Specific antibody assists the phagocytosis of these organisms. On reaching the kidney the organisms are protected against the body's defences in the renal medulla. At this stage the disease is very difficult to treat.

Depending on the species of the organism involved, the disease can vary from mild conjunctivitis to fulminating jaundice.

People at risk are those in contact with rats and contaminated water.

ACTINOMYCETES

Actinomycetes are filamentous branching organisms. The branching myce-lium is subject to fragmentation. Certain of the members of this group are saphrophytes, others are pathogenic to man.

A. MICROAEROPHILIC TO ANAEROBIC ACTINOMYCETES

These are non acid-fast organisms characterized by branching filaments.

Actinomyces israelii

Source: This organism is a commensal in the mouth. Human infections by *Actinomyces israelii* are endogenous and often preceded by trauma to the oral mucosa.

Disease Pattern: The classical lesion in actinomycosis is that of a mass. These woody masses may break down and form abscesses. Pus may be discharged by sinus formation. The pus contains 'sulphur granules'. These granules are clusters of the organism.

There are three typical clinical sites in which actinomycosis is found: 60% of cases occur in the cervico-facial region, 22% are found in the abdomen and the remainder are found in the thorax.

Treatment: Penicillin is the drug of choice. Surgical drainage is an adjunct to antibiotic therapy.

B.   AEROBIC ACTINOMYCETES

(i)   *Norcardia asteroides*

Source: Norcardia is present in soil.

Disease Pattern: The primary lesion is in the lungs. A chronic suppura-tive pulmonary lesion is usually associated with spread of the orga-nism to the central nervous system and the intestinal tract. Sinuses may form but no granules are found in the exuded pus. Norcardio-sis frequently complicates leukaemia, Hodgkin's disease or any condition associated with impaired immunity.

Treatment: Treatment in the early stages with sulphonamides or ampi-cillin may be curative.

(ii)   *Norcardia madurae*

Source: The organisms are commonly found in soil or on vegetable matter.

Disease Pattern: Infection is often preceded by trauma leading to inocu-lation of the organism. Mycetoma, often a localized lesion, starts as a papule which may become a fixed nodule or break down to form an abscess with discharging sinuses. Granules consisting of micro-colonies of norcardia are found in the discharged fluid.

Treatment: Antibiotics are useful, e.g. sulphanomides are frequently used.

Actinomycetoma must be distinguished from maduramycetoma. Clinically the lesions are similar but maduramycetoma is caused by a true fungus and treatment is with antifungal agents.

MYCOPLASMA

Mycoplasmas are simple unicellular organisms which differ from the eubacteria in lacking a cell wall. Bacteria which normally have cell walls may, on occasion, lose these cell walls — these bacteria are termed L forms or protoplasts. Protoplasts and mycoplasma have certain features in common.

(i) These organisms are resistant to penicillin. Penicillin acts on cell wall synthesis.

(ii) These organisms are susceptible to lysis due to changes in osmotic pressure.

Protoplasts are derived from bacteria — these cell wall defective mutants can occur spontaneously or be induced by chemicals. They may revert back to their bacterial form. Mycoplasmas are not derived from bacteria but form a special group of small prokaryotic organisms.

Source: Many species of mycoplasma are included amongst the normal flora and the genito-urinary tract of the oropharynx.

Disease Pattern: Disease attributed to mycoplasma organisms involve mucous membranes. The organism attaches to the cells of the mucous membrane by a plate-like appendage. Mycoplasmas are known to cause primary atypical pneumonia; they are suspected of playing a role in many diseases of the genito-urinary tract, e.g. non-gonococcal urethritis, infertility, cervicitis, etc.

Mycoplasma pneumoniae

Spread: The organism is spread by droplet inhalation.

Disease Pattern: *Mycoplasma pneumoniae* is the pathogen responsible for primary atypical pneumonia. This respiratory disease is characterized by more severe X-ray findings than are suggested on physical examination.

Treatment: Tetracycline is the drug of choice.

OBLIGATE INTRACELLULAR PARASITES

There are four groups of intracellular parasites of medical importance.

These are: The Rickettsiae (with the exception of *R. quintana*)
Coxiella burneti
The Chlamydiae
The Viruses

The first groups are prokaryotic cells, i.e. they are bacteria-like. The last group forms a group on its own. The above organisms are all located inside their host's cells. This 'anatomical' situation is not by chance — it is essential for the survival of these organisms that they infect cells. They may depend on the host cell for energy, for the correct osmotic environment or for the necessary mechanical equipment to synthesise proteins. These are obligate intracellular parasites.

THE RICKETTSIAE

Source and Spread: Lice, fleas and ticks are the common arthropod hosts involved in the transmission of rickettsial diseases. The rickettsiae are intestinal parasites of these blood sucking arthropods. They do not cause disease in their natural arthropod host.

Rickettsiae may be transmitted from arthropod to arthropod by feeding on the same infected vertebrate host or by transovarial transmission, e.g. in ticks.

Rickettsiae are transmitted to man with the assistance of the arthropod host — the organism may be transmitted in the bite of a tick or scratched into the skin defect along with the faeces of the louse. Rickettsiae enter man by way of a skin lesion created by the biting arthropod host.

Disease Pattern: The diseases caused by rickettsiae are characterized by an incubation period of 7-10 days. The rickettsiae parasitize endothelial cells. The organisms multiply in the host cell by means of binary fission and appear to have little effect on the host cell. When sufficient multiplication has occurred, the host cell, now packed with rickettsiae, bursts. The released rickettsiae seek new host cells. Entry into the host cell is an active process requiring the use of energy in the form of ATP (adenosine triphosphate). The target cell of the rickettsial infection is the endothelial cell of blood vessels — rickettsia cause vascular infections. The local lesion may be referred to as the typhus node.

The host's response to rickettsial infection is usually associated with fever and a rash. The presence of infected endothelial cells in the central nervous systems vasculature can be associated with delirium. Infected endothelial cells in the pulmonary blood vessels can present as pneumonitis.

Different species of rickettsiae are transmitted by different arthropod hosts and are associated with different clinical diseases.

Table XXVIII

RICKETTSIAE TRANSMITTED TO MAN

THE ORGANISM	ARTHROPOD HOST	DISEASE IN MAN
R. prowazeki	louse	Epidemic typhus
R. mooseri	flea	Murine (Endemic) typhus
R. conori	tick	Tick bite fever
R. akari	mite	Rickettsial pox
R. rickettsiae	tick	Rocky mountain spotted fever
R. tsutsugamushi	mite	Scrub typhus

Treatment: Tetracycline is the drug of choice. Administration of tetracyclines is necessary for a full 48 hours before a clinical response
is detected.

Rickettsiae are prokaryotic cells with thick cell walls and contain both
DNA and RNA.

Coxiella Burneti

Coxiella burneti differs from rickettsiae in that they are stable outside host
cells; rickettsiae have unstable leaky cell membranes. These organisms
were previously classified amongst the rickettsiae.

Source and Spread: This agent may be spread by ticks, but it is more
often spread in dust. Aerosol spread from animal products and
contaminated dust are important sources of infection. The fine dust
layer covering the hide of a goat, a cow or a sheep may harbour
this organism.

Disease Pattern: *Coxiella burneti* causes Q fever. Q fever has the fever
common to the rickettsial diseases; it does not, however, have the
characteristic skin rash. Q fever is characterized by respiratory and
hepatic symptoms.

Treatment: Tetracycline is the drug of choice. Coxiella are less susceptible to tetracycline than rickettsiae.

Chlamydiae

Chlamydiae contain both DNA and RNA. They have their own 70s ribosomes and do not depend on their host's cell machinery for protein synthesis. They are energy parasites. Chlamydiae lack the full complement of
cytochromes. A defective electron ladder leads to defective ATP production. Chlamydiae depend on the host cell for ATP. Chlamydiae are more
dependent than rickettsiae for metabolic aid from their host cell.

The infectious chlamydial particle is termed the 'elementary body'.
Elementary bodies are phagocytosed by the host cell. Once inside the host
cell, surrounded by the host cell's cytoplasmic membrane, the chlamydial
organism is reorganised and an 'initial body' is formed. Multiplication of
the organism by binary fission leads to the formation of 'inclusion bodies'.
These inclusion bodies may be liberated and new cells can become infected.
The chlamydial cycle takes 24-48 hours.

There are two groups of chlamydiae —

(*a*) those which cause psittacosis;

(*b*) those responsible for the trachoma — lymphogranuloma venereum
complex of diseases.

In their natural hosts chlamydiae produce subclinical rather than overt
infection.

Psittacosis

Source: This is a disease of birds. The organism may be transferred to
man.

Spread: *Chlamydia psittici* is spread by inhalation of the excreta of infected birds.

Disease Pattern: Psittacosis is associated with headache, fever and a pneumonitis-like picture. Respiratory symptoms are prominent. Organs of the reticulo-endothelial system — the lungs, liver and spleen are all infected. The mortality rate may be as high as 20%.

Treatment: Tetracyclines are used in the treatment of psittacosis. They are unable to prevent the carrier state.

Trachoma-lymphogranuloma venereum complex

Source and Spread: These chalmydiae are probably spread from man to man by direct contact, or by indirect contact — eye to finger to eye or genitalia to finger to eye.

Disease Pattern: These chlamydiae are responsible for both ocular and genital infections in man. The eye involvement varies from trachoma, a condition leading to blindness, to inclusion conjunctivitis, a condition producing minimal corneal scarring.

Lymphogranuloma venereum is a venereal disease which in the chronic stages is characterized by excessive fibrosis, scarring, stricture formation and lymphatic obstruction. The lymphadenopathy of early lymphogranuloma venereum, unlike that of syphilis, is painful.

Treatment: Sulphonamides are the drugs of choice in the treatment in the trachoma-lymphogranuloma complex.

VIRUSES

These agents differ from the other obligate intracellular parasites in certain important respects:

  (i) Viruses contain either DNA or RNA, not both. Exceptions to this rule include variola.

  (ii) They do not multiply by binary fission.

  (iii) They undergo an 'eclipse' phase during infection of the host cell. During this period the virus is indistinguishable from the constituents of the host cell.

  (iv) They are completely dependent on the host cell for the machinery and raw materials necessary for life and replication. Viruses possess the blue print — the host supplies the factory.

The infectious viral particle is termed a virion. A virion consists of a central core of nucleic acid, either DNA or RNA, protected by a protein coat, the capsid. Together the protein coat and the nucleic acid constitute the nucleocapsid. Certain viruses have an outer membrane called the envelope surrounding the nucleocapsid. The envelope is partly derived from the host's cell membrane.

Viruses are spread from patients, carriers and from healthy individuals who are in the incubation stage of the disease. Viruses are spread by droplets, by contact, venereally, by congenital spread and by arthropods.

Viruses may be ingested, inhaled or introduced through a lesion in the skin or mucous membranes. As these organisms require the host cell's machinery for their replication, it is necessary for them to enter the cell and establish themselves in an intracellular environment.

Infection of the host cell by the virion starts with the adsorption phase. Contact between the virus and the host cell leads to adsorption, provided the proteins of the virus have a specific affinity for the receptor site on that host cell. The protein coat of the virus is antigenic and stimulates antibody production in the host. Specific antibody can inhibit adsorption of the virus onto the host cell.

Penetration of the virus into the cytoplasm of the host cell is accompanied by the loss of the viral envelope. The virus then undergoes a process of uncoating at the end of which the nucleic acid of the virus is lying free in the host cell.

The viral nucleic acid now directs cell metabolism to produce viral nucleic acid, enzymes and proteins. During this phase the virus is not detectable within the cell. The 'eclipse' phase ends with the assembly of these constituents into new virus particles. Viral assembly may take place in either the nucleus or the cytoplasm of the host cell. The infected cell may lyse and release the virions or these may bud off from the cell cytoplasmic membrane.

In summary, viruses infect host cells in the following sequence:
  (i) Adsorption — the virus attaches to the host cell membrane.
  (ii) Pinocytosis — the virus moves from outside (extracellular) to the inside (intracellular) of the host cell.
  (iii) Uncoating — the virus loses its covering and lies naked as the nucleic acid.
  (iv) Eclipse phase — viral replication takes place. The constituents of the virus are not distinguishable from host cell constituents.
  (v) Assembly — the viral constituents are assembled into virus particles.

The virus may effect the host cell in a number of ways —
  (*a*) It may cause histological changes in the cell, e.g. giant cells may be formed as in infections with the respiratory syncitial virus; inclusion bodies may be formed in either the nucleus or the cytoplasm, e.g. herpes or poxviruses. These inclusions may be altered host cells or viral particle aggregates.
  (*b*) It may cause physiological changes in the cell, e.g. rubella leads to decreased cell growth and multiplication; papilloma virus leads to increased cell proliferation.

Viral-host cell interaction may fall into one of three possible patterns:
  (1) The lytic cycle. When a virulent virus infects a cell it utilizes that cell as a factory for its (the virus') reproduction. The cell bursts or

Figure 22
INFECTION OF AN ANIMAL CELL BY A VIRUS

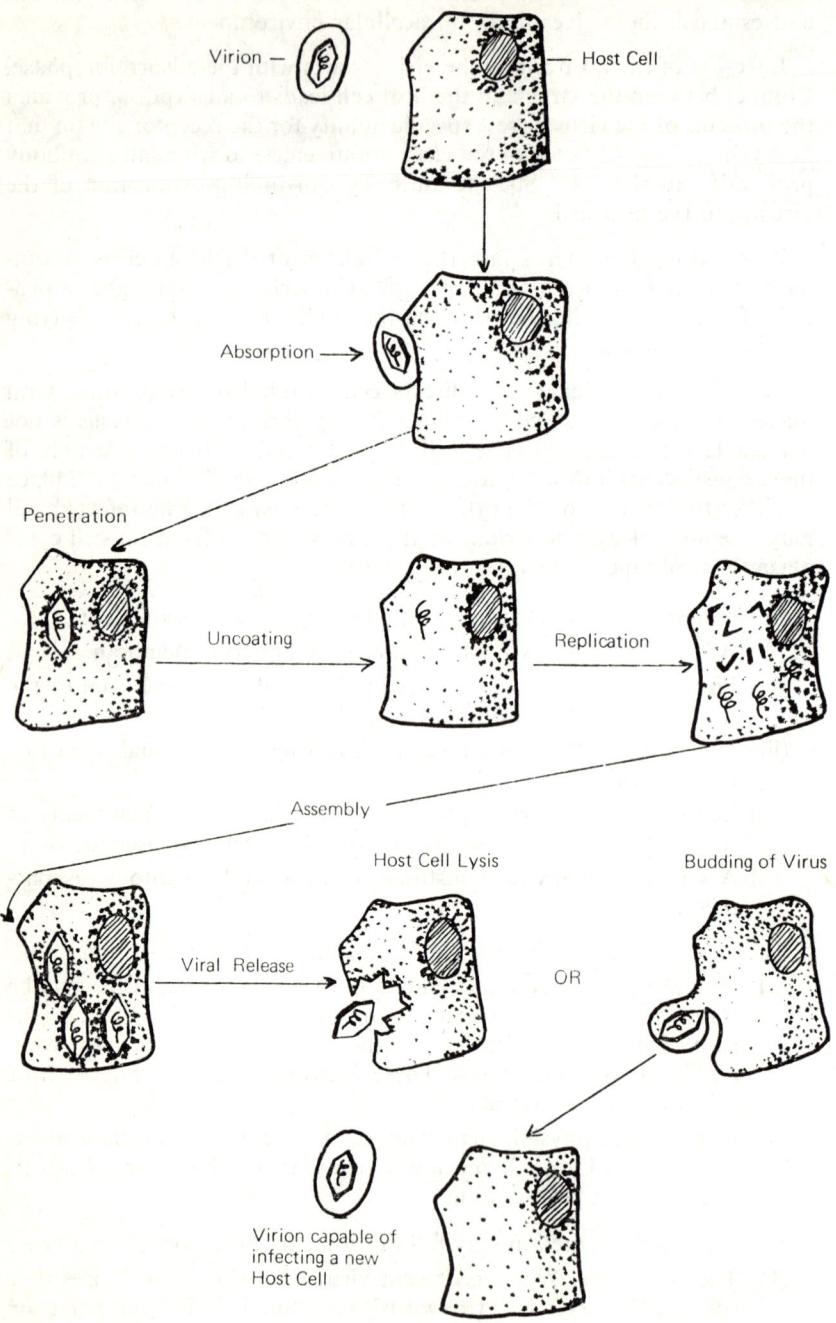

Virion —

Host Cell

Absorption →

Penetration

Uncoating

Replication

Assembly

Host Cell Lysis

Budding of Virus

Viral Release →

OR

Virion capable of
infecting a new
Host Cell

lyses when replication of the virus is complete. The released viruses are then capable of infecting new cells and repeating the cycle.

(2) A steady state cycle. The virus and host cell live in equilibrium. The virus does not lyse the cell, instead the cell steadily and slowly releases the new viruses produced within its cytoplasm and/or nucleus.

(3) Lysogeny. Lysogeny is an infection of a cell in which the virus does not propagate except in synchronomy with the host's cell chromosomes. Virions are not produced. Host cells may acquire certain new characteristics as a result of this interaction with the viral nucleic acid. Examples of lysogenic conversion amongst bacteria infected by viruses include the ability bestowed on *C. diphtheriae* to produce diphtheria toxin, and upon *Streptococcus pyogenes* to produce erythrogenic toxin.

The virus may leave the host cell by budding off from the host cell or it may be released by lysis of the host cell. The shed virus then spreads and infects other cells. Spread to other cells may be by direct contact, by spread in natural passages, by blood spread or in lymphocytes. Virus may also be released into the environment and infect others.

When a virus infects a new host it undergoes a period of multiplication. This is the incubation period, which is an asymptomatic period starting with the infection of a host and ending with the appearance of the first symptom. The incubation for many of the common viral infections, e.g. measles, mumps, rubella and chicken-pox, varies between one and two or three weeks. Multiplication at the site of the primary focus can lead to spread of the virus in the host — virus may also be shed into the environment. The spread of the virus, often inside macrophages, into lymphatics and via the thoracic duct into the blood stream, leads to the primary viraemia. The primary viraemia is manifest clinically as the prodromal signs or as the minor illness.

In general there are two different kinds of clinical presentations in viral diseases. The first is characterized by a biphasic illness — the minor illness followed by the major illness. Viruses multiply at the site of introduction, i.e. local multiplication occurs; this is followed by systemic spread. During and after the primary viraemia, macrophages of the reticulo-endothelial system phagocytose the viruses. After the minor illness further viral multiplication occurs followed by a secondary viraemia with spread of the virus to target organs. The major illness is the latter phase of the disease. The individual may acquire life-long immunity after his initial illness. The time delay between the minor and major illness in subsequent infections gives the host the opportunity to produce antibodies or re-stimulate his primed cell mediated immunity. The antibody produced neutralises virus during the second viraemic phase and prevents viral infection of the target organs.

The second classical viral disease pattern is that of local and systemic clinical symptoms in the absence of systemic viral spread. In the absence of viraemia, immunity is short lived. This is especially true of viruses subject to frequent antigenic alteration, e.g. influenza.

Host defences against viral infections involve both humoral and cellular immune mechanisms. Antibodies neutralize the virus and prevent attachment of the virus to the host cell. Viruses which are unable to infect cells are incapable of replication. Neutralized virus, while unable to attach to target cells and cause disease, is more easily phagocytosed by cells of the immune system. The cell mediated immune system produces cytotoxic cells capable of killing the virus. These killer cells play an important role in immunity to viral infections. Primed lymphocytes also produce a humoral substance, interferon, which prevents multiplication of the virus. Interferon production interferes with viral protein synthesis. Interferon is produced early in infection — in fact it precedes antibody production.

Viruses can infect any organ system. Many viruses have specific target organs, e.g. the skin in the case of herpes I and III; mucous membranes in the case of herpes II; the respiratory tract in the case of the influenza viruses and the nervous system in the case of rabies and poliomyelitis. The liver bears the brunt of infection in yellow fever and in both serum and infectious hepatitis. During the primary viraemia many viruses are removed by platelets, lymphocytes and monocytes, and killed; those that are not removed and killed reach their target organs. Measles and rubella both start as infections of the respiratory tract. They both spread systemically and present clinically as skin rashes. Occasionally the portal of entry and the target organ are the same, e.g. influenza.

Viruses may give rise to a clinical syndrome which is characteristic of that virus, e.g. smallpox, or they may present clinically as manifestations of organ dysfunction. Many different viruses may thus give a similar clinical picture when the feature of the disease is that of organ dysfunction, e.g. aseptic meningitis. This broad pattern of organism specific disease is also found amongst bacterial infections.

Slow virus infections

Certain viruses or certain altered viruses are capable of causing slow viral infections. Slow viral disease may follow clinical or subclinical infections. They are characterized by long incubation periods, e.g. years. Different slow virus diseases may be accompanied by one or more of the following features: demyelination, immune complex disease or spongioform degeneration. Subacute sclerosing panencephalitis occurs in people who have all had measles. The measles virus or an altered measles virus is believed to cause the disease in certain individuals. Subacute sclerosing panencephalitis occurs years after the acute attack of measles.

Workers feel that certain agents even smaller than viruses may be incriminated in the aetiology of disease at present classified as slow virus diseases. Amongst these is the agent responsible for Kuru. The membrane bound agent responsible for Kuru is not believed to be antigenic. It causes disease by its persistent multiplication in the host cell. After several years the agent is believed to cause degeneration of the infected host cells. Kuru was first described as a disease confined to females in a certain tribe. The females in this tribe had the custom of eating their deceased grandmother's brain. The grandmothers had terminated with Kuru — an illness characterized by central nervous system degeneration. Infection of the female members of the tribe occurred by ingestion of the infected brain. The males escaped Kuru as they ingested the tastier muscles of grandmother.

The classification of viruses

Viruses can be classified into two large groups on the basis of their nucleic acid. Further differentiation on the presence or absence of an envelope is made. Enveloped viruses are sensitive to ether and bile; viruses not enveloped are resistant to these substances. Virions are sensitive to phenols and ultraviolet light; they are stabilized in salt solutions.

Table XXIX
A CLASSIFICATION OF VIRUSES

DNA VIRUSES
DNA viruses with envelopes
    Double stranded enveloped DNA viruses —
        Herpesviruses
        Poxviruses

DNA viruses without an envelope
    Double stranded naked DNA viruses —
        Papova virus
        Adenovirus
    Single stranded DNA viruses —
        Parvovirus

RNA VIRUSES
RNA viruses with envelopes
    Single stranded enveloped RNA viruses —
        Orthomyxoviruses   — influenza
        Paramyxoviruses   — parainfluenza
                      — measles
                      — mumps
                      — respiratory syncitial
      Togaviruses (formally classified amongst the arboviruses)
      Rhabdovirus

RNA viruses without envelopes
    Naked single stranded RNA viruses —
        Picorna viruses —   (*a*) Rhinovirus
                    (*b*) Enterovirus — poliovirus
                                          — coxsackievirus
                                        — echovirus

    Naked double stranded RNA viruses —
        Reovirus
    Other RNA viruses —
        Coronavirus

UNCLASSIFIED
The viruses responsible for infective and serum hepatitis have not yet been fully classified.

THE ARBOVIRUSES

This is a group of viruses grouped together on the basis of their mode of transmission. All the above viruses are transmitted by arthropods. Arboviruses are further classified into the following groups —

alphaviruses $\Big\}$ Togaviruses
flaviviruses
rhabdoviruses
orbiviruses
bunyaviruses

A CONSIDERATION OF CERTAIN MEDICALLY IMPORTANT VIRUSES

THE DNA VIRUSES

The herpes group of viruses

This group of viruses is characterized by latent infection and clinical recurrences. They are also postulated to play a role in certain malignant diseases in man and animals. There are five members of the herpes family known to cause disease in man.

Herpes type I   — *Herpesvirus homonis*/herpes labialis
Herpes type II   — *Herpesvirus genitalis*
Herpes type III — *Herpesvirus varicella*
Herpes type IV   — Ebstein Barr virus
Herpes type V   — Cytomegalovirus

Herpes type I

Primary infection with herpes I leads to gingivo-stomatitis.

Source and Spread: Man is the source of *Herpesvirus hominis*. The virus is secreted in the saliva and may be spread directly or by contamination of fomites with infected saliva.

Pathogenesis: Herpes type I is adapted to the head and neck region. It infects cells and undergoes a lytic cycle leading to rupture of the cell with vesicle formation. The vesicle ulcerates to leave a painful base. The virus spreads in the same individual by continuity and contiguity.

Recrudescence of herpes labialis is common. The precipitating factor may be stress — emotional or physical, sunlight or a feverish illness. No precipitating factor need be apparent.

Clinical Disease: The common manifestation of herpes I is as a vesicle which breaks down to form a white ulcer with a red rim. Lips are most commonly involved — tongue, gums and conjunctiva may also be involved.

Most individuals (50-98 %) are infected with herpes by the age of five years. Recurrences occur in less than half this number; recurrence of herpes conjunctivitis can lead to herpes kerato-conjunctivitis and blindness.

A rare but serious complication of herpes type I infection is herpes encephalitis. This condition usually leads to death or mental retardation. Treatment with nucleic acid analogues is of limited value.

Herpes type II

Source and Spread: Herpes type II or herpes genitalis is spread by direct contact. The virus is spread by venereal contact. The primary lesion is usually on the penis, the vagina or the cervix.

Clinical Disease: The lesion of herpes genitalis is similar to that of herpes type I. A painful herpes ulcer can lead to dysparunia (painful intercourse) for the afflicted partner.

Infection of the baby as it passes down the birth canal can lead to neonatal herpes. Neonatal herpes varies from mild to severe generalized disease. It is best avoided by caesarean section. Herpes type II may or may not be an aetiological factor in cervical cancer. Those women who present with cervical cancer of a particular histological type have a high correlation rate with frequent sexual intercourse, a variety of partners, trichononiasis, syphilis and herpes II.

The incidence of herpes genitalis is very low below the age of 10 years. The incidence then increases. The prevalence of the disease varies in different population groups; in certain groups it is as high as 80%. Like herpes I, herpes II recurs at intervals.

Herpes type III

Source and Spread: Chicken-pox is a highly infectious condition that spreads by droplets or contact with the skin lesions. It is usually acquired in childhood.

Disease pattern: The skin is the target organ for varicella. Papules, vesicles, and ulcers covered by scabs occur in crops. The trunk is the area mainly involved.

Chicken-pox, a mild disease in children, must be distinguished from smallpox. Both are spread by droplets, both present with papules, vesicles and scab covered ulcers. The lesions in chicken-pox are mainly on the trunk; those of smallpox have a peripheral distribution. The lesions in chicken-pox are found at different stages of development; those of smallpox are all at the same stage. Chicken-pox is caused by a herpes virus, smallpox by a poxvirus.

Herpes zoster

This is a recrudescent herpes. The virus causes painful vesicles and ulcers in the distribution of the nerve roots. Zoster found on the trunk is attributed to varicella, that on the face to herpes type I and that in the genital region to herpes III.

Zoster occurs in adults. The virus is thought to be latent in the dorsal root ganglion of the nerve supplying the dermatome which develops the lesion. Contact spread of zoster is rare.

Herpes type IV

Disease Pattern: Infectious mononucleosis or glandular fever is due to
an infection by the Ebstein-Barr virus (EB virus), herpes group IV.
This disease presents as a sore throat accompanied by generalized
enlargement of the reticulo-endothelial system (spleen and lymph
nodes particularly), and a lymphocytosis.

Infectious mononucleosis is an interrupted malignancy of the lymph-
glands — lymphocytes infected by the EB virus multiply and are capable
of forming cell lines. Lymphocytes not infected by this virus behave as
normal cells and are incapable of producing cell lines. A characteristic of
malignant cells is their ability to form cell lines.

The EB virus may play an aetiological role in the evolution of a tumour
of the jaw. Burkitts lymphoma, and also nasopharyngeal carcinoma, are
primarily diseases found in African children.

Herpes type V

Cytomegalovirus or herpes type V is a virus well adapted to man. Most
infections are subclinical. Once infected, man probably carries the latent
virus for life.

Cytomegalovirus can cause severe disease in the foetus. A mother who
acquires the disease during pregnancy can spread the virus transplacentally
to her unborn child. Infection during the third trimester leads to infection
of all the foetus's parenchymal organs except muscle and bone. The disease
can lead to death of the infected foetus, those babies that survive have
hepatic, haematological and central nervous system defects.

Immunity and the herpes group of viruses

Herpes types I, III and V are especially of interest in patients who are
subject to immunosuppression. Immunosuppressed patients can develop
fatal generalized disease due to recrudescence of latent infections by these
viruses.

The poxviruses

The target organ in infections with the poxvirus is the skin. Different poxviruses infect man and animals. Variola is the poxvirus responsible for
smallpox. In 1967 smallpox was endemic in 30 communities. The WHO
undertook an extensive eradication campaign and in 1975 announced the
global eradication of this disease. In late 1976 further cases of smallpox
were diagnosed in Somalia. This disease can be fatal and travellers require
vaccination against smallpox on moving from one country to another.
The vaccine used to protect against smallpox consists of a live attenuated
vaccinia virus. The vaccinia and variola viruses have antigenic similarities.

The adenoviruses

Adenoviruses preferentially infect mucous membrane surfaces. They spread
from person to person; the incidence of adenovirus infection increases
rapidly in susceptible populations when overcrowding is present.

Adenovirus infection leads to acute upper and lower respiratory tract infection. Infection with one of the adenovirus strains leads to a whooping cough-like syndrome. Adenovirus is also a cause of conjunctivitis.

Adenovirus may persist for years in lymphoid tissue.

The papovavirus group
Papovaviruses usually cause disease in animals. One member of the group causes warts in man.

The parvoviruses
Members of this group are believed to cause diarrhoea in man.

THE RNA VIRUSES
The picornaviruses
Amongst this group are two subgroups important to man. These are:

(*a*) The enteroviruses

(*b*) The rhinoviruses

The rhinovirus group are the viruses most commonly implicated as the cause of the common cold. Spread is by droplet infection.

The enteroviruses
Spread of the enteroviruses is faecal-oral. Good hygiene may therefore play an important role in decreasing their spread. Members of the enterovirus group include —

> The poliovirus
> The coxsachieviruses } these cause important diseases.

The echovirus is responsible for aseptic meningitis. Echovirus may also cause a rash which may or may not be accompanied by fever. The echovirus has been incriminated as a cause of the common cold.

Enterovirus 70 causes acute haemorrhage conjunctivitis.

Hepatitis A, the virus causing infective hepatitis, is probably a picornavirus.

The poliovirus
The poliovirus is spread by the faecal-oral route. Ingestion of the virus leads to multiplication of the virus in the lymphoid tissue of the throat and intestinal tract.

Clinically, most infections with the poliovirus are sub-clinical. Overt infections may present as a minor illness with a sore throat, fever, anorexia and headache. These symptoms last a few days. Abortive polio stops after the minor illness, paralytic polio proceeds to the major illness where muscle pain and paralysis become major symptoms. The poliovirus destroys the motor neurones.

Poliovirus may occasionally be detected in the patient's stool for up to six months after the onset of clinical symptoms. The most infectious period is, however, during the minor illness. Virus is also present in the patient's throat during the early stages of the disease. By the time the child presents with paralysis it is difficult to isolate the virus.

Polio can be successfully prevented by adequate immunization. The live attenuated virus used in the polio vaccine can be differentiated from the wild strain in the laboratory.

The coxsackieviruses

Coxsackieviruses are divided into two groups. A number of different clinical syndromes have been attributed to these viruses.

Coxsackie A

This viral infection presents with fever, rash and/or meningoencephalitis. One or more of these symptoms may be present in the patient simultaneously.

Coxsackie B

This virus may present a similar clinical picture to coxsackie A. Coxsackie B is also associated with pleurodynia (severe pleuritic pain) in the adult. It may be the cause of fatal myocarditis in the neonate.

Coxsackie B infections are especially common amongst children. Children are not permitted to visit mothers in maternity hospitals. Coxsackie B is one of the reasons for this restriction. Outbreaks of coxsackie B myocarditis in maternity hospitals have led to the closing of that hospital.

The arenaviruses

Included in the arenavirus group is Lassa fever virus. Lassa fever is an often fatal disease spread by this highly contagious virus. In the absence of extreme precautions in the examination and nursing of these patients, infection of the nursing and medical attendants is a serious hazard. Gloves, masks, complete change of clothing, caps and goggles are recommended in the safe handling of Lassa fever cases.

Slow viruses are also grouped amongst the arenaviruses.

The orthomyxoviruses

Influenzavirus

This virus has three different types — influenzavirus A, B and C. Influenza type A is responsible for epidemics, type B is endemic. All the influenza viruses are subject to frequent antigenic alteration. It is, therefore, possible to have many attacks of influenza in one lifetime. Influenza may herald the start of a terminal illness for the elderly cardiac or respiratory cripple. Every year the employer will lose a substantial number of working hours due to staff illness caused by the influenzavirus. Influenza is thus an economic hazard in the healthy individual. It may sound the death knell for the elderly.

The paramyxoviruses

Parainfluenza

These viruses infect the respiratory tract. There are four different types —

type I causes lower respiratory disease; type II causes upper respiratory disease and type III causes both. Type IV does not cause human disease. Laryngo-tracheo bronchitis and croup are important diseases caused by the parainfluenza viruses.

Respiratory syncitial virus

These paramyxoviruses are responsible for respiratory diseases during childhood.

Rubeolavirus

Measles starts as a catarrhal illness. During this stage the virus is rapidly spread by droplets. In a susceptible population one individual with measles may infect four others. Measles is more infectious than influenza.

Measles is usually diagnosed when the fever, cough and runny nose are improving and the maculopapular rash appears. Secondary bacterial infection of the respiratory tract is a problem. Bacterial complications in measles include broncho-pneumonia, otitis media, chronic sinusitis and blindness. The incidence of bacterial complications of measles increases in direct proportion to the degree of malnutrition, and poor socio-economic circumstances of the victims.

Measles may be complicated by encephalitis in any population group. Measles or an altered measles virus appears responsible for a slow virus disease.

Paramyxovirus parotidis — the mumps virus

Mumps, like measles, is a common contagious disease of childhood. Spread is by droplet infection. The target organs in mumps are the salivary glands, notably the parotid, the pancreas and the gonads. Adult males may become sterile after an attack of mumps orchitis.

Newcastle Disease

This is a disease of fowls caused by a RNA virus. Men working with sick chickens can develop Newcastle conjunctivitis.

The togaviruses

Rubella

The virus responsible for German measles is included in this group. Spread of rubella is by droplets from the respiratory tract. Infection leads to the development of a rash and occipital lymphadenopathy. German measles in the mature individual is a mild disease. Foetal infection with rubella-virus may lead to the congenital rubella syndrome. When expectant mothers are infected during the first or even in the second trimester of pregnancy the virus spreads transplacentally and infects the foetus. The virus infects the cells of the developing foetus and slows down cell multiplication. Infected foetuses may be born with a variety of different clinical symptoms, e.g. blindness, deafness, heart defects, etc.

Many arboviruses are grouped amongst the togaviruses.

Coronaviruses

These viruses cause acute upper respiratory tract infections.

Rhabdoviruses

Marburg and rabies viruses both fall into this category. They are animal viruses which may cause fatal disease in man.

Rabies virus is spread in the saliva of infected animals. Rabies is spread by meercats, dogs and many other wild animals. All these animals are sick and often die. The natural host of rabies may be the bat. Rabies is not known to spread from man to man. It causes spasm of the neck and throat muscles and this has earned it the name of hydrophobia. Rabies effects the nervous system — excitation and paralysis precede death.

Reovirus group

These viruses may cause diarrhoea in man.

Arboviruses

The arboviruses are grouped together on the basis of their mode of transmission. All the arboviruses are transmitted by arthropods. The arthropods commonly incriminated are ticks and mosquitoes. Arboviruses often have a wide range of possible vertebrate hosts. The distribution of arboviruses depends on the presence of the arthropod and the presence of the vertebrate host.

Important diseases amongst this group are yellow fever, dengue, chickungunye, rift valley fever and west nile. Arboviruses are also responsible for a number of different encephalitis syndromes.

Unclassified

Hepatitis B

This virus is responsible for serum hepatitis. Australia antigen, the Dane particle and long incubation hepatitis virus, are all different names for this virus.

The virus is spread in the blood or in blood products, in saliva and in seminal fluid. It may give rise to an acute disease which may result in recovery or lead to chronic liver disease. Sub-clinical disease followed by a carrier state is common in certain population groups, e.g. the rural African.

Rotavirus

This virus is a cause of gastro-enteritis in babies.

TREATMENT

Viral infections are widespread. The treatment of viral infections is for the most part symptomatic. Specific therapy is difficult as the action of the drug must be directed against the viral nucleic acid. Viral and host nucleic acid are structurally composed of very similar building blocks. Any agent used to specifically treat a viral infection will have toxic side effects. Only individuals with critical viral diseases are thus considered as candidates for specific therapy. Herpes encephalitis, a condition, which when not fatal leaves the victim mentally retarded, is treated with a drug which interferes with nucleic acid metabolism. Hyper-immune gamma globulin is occasionally used but this must be administered early in the diseases before the virus has attached to its target organ.

Non-specific therapy, such as adequate nutrition, treatment of acute respiratory obstruction with tracheostomy or intubation are all important adjuncts in the treatment of viral diseases. Bed rest and anti-pyretics are often the only treatments available. Prevention and treatment of secondary bacterial infections, especially secondary bacterial pneumonias, may be life saving.

CHAPTER 5

Organ Systems and Disease

Clinical syndromes can be determined by the type of infecting organism or the site of the infection:

(*a*) The clinical picture can be characteristic of the infecting organism. Exotoxin producing organisms are those that present with a clinical picture dictated by the organism. Tetanus is a disease presenting with muscle spasms and convulsions due to the effects of tetanospasmin on the nervous system. Botulism is characterized by paralysis, a direct result of the ingestion of botulinum toxin. The pattern of the disease can be indicative of the causative organism, e.g. diphtheria is a clinical diagnosis only later confirmed by the laboratory.

(*b*) Infection can be diagnosed on the basis of organ dysfunction, e.g. meningitis, gastro-enteritis, salpingitis, cystitis. Infection of an organ system by any one of a multitude of organisms can give a similar clinical picture. Each organ system has only a limited range of responses, e.g. cystitis manifests as an irritable bladder — the motor activity of the bladder is increased resulting in frequency; the sensory component registers an altered urine — burning on micturition is therefore common in cystitis. Frequency, urgency and burning are diagnostic of cystitis. The organism responsible for the cystitis could be an *E. coli*, a proteus, a klebsiella, a *Strept. faecalis* or many other bacteria. Regardless of the species or even if more than one species of bacterium is responsible, the clinical picture and diagnosis remains the same. The diagnosis of cystitis depends on the bladder's expression of dysfunction, not on the type of infecting organism. Pneumonia is lung dysfunction — this is clinically demonstrated by dyspnoea, chest pain and a productive cough. Different bacteria — pneumococcus, klebsiella, staphylococcus and other bacteria causing pneumonia give a similar picture.

All infections do have one sign in common. Fever is usually present when there is an imbalance in the host-parasite equilibrium. The presence of fever is, however, not pathognomonic of infection. Fever may also be present in non-infective conditions, e.g. the collagen diseases, cancer, Hodgkin's disease.

THE RESPIRATORY SYSTEM

Approximately one quarter of the general practitioner's working life is spent treating respiratory diseases. Infection of the respiratory system accounts for about one third of absenteeism from work. The main cause of this absenteeism is attributable to upper respiratory tract infections.

The respiratory tract starts at the nose and passes through the pharynx down the trachea, bronchi and bronchioles to end in the alveoli. This whole system is adapted to making air and thus oxygen available to the blood, the erythrocytes, and therefore to the whole body. The inhaled air is moistened, warmed and filtered by the respiratory system. Air passing through the nose develops turbulent flow due to the structure of the turbinate bones. Air turbulence brings particles into contact with the mucous coat. The nose has a normal flora. Included in this flora are corynebacteria, staphylococci and streptococci. These organisms when carried by the medical staff constitute a danger in neonatal, burns and surgical units. Nasopharyngeal carriage of pneumococci (30% of people) and *Neisseria meningitidis* (carrier rate increases from 5% to 90% in over-crowded conditions) can represent a serious hazard to hospitalized patients.

The respiratory tract below the level of the epiglottis is normally sterile. At birth the pharynx, trachea and bronchi are sterile; within 24 hours after birth these passages are colonized by α-haemolytic streptococci and nonpathogenic neisseria.

The respiratory tract is well endowed with physical and chemical components of the superficial defence barrier. The sneeze reflex expels particles from the nose; the cough reflex expels particles from the respiratory tract. In the nose the nasal hairs trap large particles; in the remainder of the respiratory tract the $5\,\mu$ thick carpet of mucus traps smaller particles. The particles adhering to the mucus layer are moved to the pharynx by the escalator action of the mucus on the rhythmically beating cilia. Mucus reaching the pharynx is either expectorated or swallowed. The physiological movement of the bronchi also encourages the movement of mucus into the trachea. The mucus layer is not inert but is in itself a chemical barrier, containing both specific and non-specific anti-microbial substances. Glycoproteins can neutralize virus particles preventing adherence to cells; lysozyme and transferrin exert an antibacterial action. Specific IgA is produced locally and secreted into the respiratory tract.

Infectious agents overcome the host's defences by causing excess mucus secretion thereby causing a defect in the cilial escalator. Patients with a tracheostomy are particularly liable to infection as the inhaled air is less humid than that which has been processed by the respiratory system above the tracheostomy orifice. The mucus dries. Cracks in the mucus blanket lead to defects in the cilial escalator. Patients with tracheostomies require administration of humidified air. Patients recovering from general anaesthesia have depressed cilial activity; they may also be secreting excess respiratory secretions. Patients who have had abdominal surgery are particularly loathe to cough up these excess secretions.

Particles entering the normally sterile bronchioli and alveoli are usually rapidly removed by macrophages. These particles are then transported out of the lung tissue to the draining lymphnodes.

The normal defences of the respiratory system depend upon the following factors —

(a) Mechanical factors — expulsion of matter by the cough and sneeze reflex, the upward movement of the mucus blanket on the cilial escalator, the introduction of turbulence into the air entering the respiratory system, physiological movement of the bronchi moving secretions upwards.

(b) Chemical factors — mucus containing glycoproteins.

(c) Microbial factors — the upper regions of the respiratory system have a normal bacterial population. Certain potential pathogens may, however, be part of the normal flora in a proportion of the population, e.g. staphylococci.

Humoral defences —

(i) non-specific — lysozyme, transferrin;

(ii) specific — IgA.

Cellular defences — the macrophage plays a vital role in protection of the alveolus.

The respiratory system is a frequent portal of entry for micro-organisms. The anatomical and physiological characteristics of the respiratory system permit not only the entry of organisms into the body by this route, but also provide the organism with a good mode of spread to other hosts. Inhaled air is not sterile. It contains micro-organisms plus other organic and inorganic matter. The larger particles are filtered in the upper respiratory tract and never reach the lung. The smaller particles of under $6\,\mu$ enter the lung and tend to settle in the alveoli or smaller bronchioles. Particles of less than $0,5\,\mu$ remain suspended and are exhaled. *Mycobacterium tuberculosis* is about $0,4$ by $3,0\,\mu$ in size; gram positive cocci are approximately $1,0\,\mu$ in diameter. These organisms are too large to remain suspended and be exhaled; they are too small to be prevented from entering the lower respiratory tract. Organisms are often inhaled associated with dust particles. Viruses which cause upper respiratory tract infections lead to cell damage. They can destroy cilia and stimulate hypersecretion of mucus. Interference with the muco-ciliary escalator facilitates the spread of bacteria down to the level of the alveoli. Individuals who interfere with the normal defences of their respiratory system, whether by smoking or excess alcohol consumption, all increase their risk of acquiring respiratory tract infections.

During speaking, coughing and sneezing the respiratory system functions as a potential microbial spray gun. Infected secretions are shed in the form of droplets. Large droplets of $100\,\mu$ fall rapidly to settle on the floor, on bedding, on surgical equipment, dressings, etc. *Mycobacterium tuberculosis*, *Corynebacterium diphtheriae*, streptococci, staphylococci are all bacteria which will survive for days and months in dried secretions or dust, provided they are not exposed to ultra-violet light. Dusty, shady areas may therefore harbour pathogenic micro-organisms. These organisms may be spread to new hosts by direct contact or indirectly by infected dust or fomites. The moisture in droplets of less than 100 μ evaporates and the organisms remaining do not settle but may be directly inhaled, e.g. measles, chicken-pox.

Infectious respiratory diseases are therefore spread by the expulsion of infected secretions from the respiratory system and contracted by the inhalation of infected dust or secretory droplets. Overcrowding is an important factor in the spread of bacterial respiratory infections. The incidence of viral respiratory disease is similar in all sections of the population; the incidence of bacterial respiratory disease is proportional to overcrowding and poverty. The distance between beds in institutions has been shown to be a critical factor in the spread of organisms. The carrier rate of meningococci more than doubles in army camps; this increase in the carrier rate is significantly less if the distance between beds is increased. The incidence of rheumatic fever shows a positive correlation with overcrowding — spread of *Streptococcus pyogenes* is increased under these conditions. The number of hospital beds permitted per hospital ward is influenced by the respiratory spread of disease.

Medical and nursing staff, when dealing with patients who are immunodepressed, when dressing surgical wounds, when delivering babies, or when inserting a urinary catheter, all wear masks. These masks must be worn covering both mouth and nose. The mask is an attempt on the part of the hospital staff to decrease the patient's risk of acquiring potentially pathogenic organisms from the upper respiratory tract of the attendant.

Disease of the upper respiratory tract may manifest as coryza, pharyngitis, laryngitis, tracheitis or croup. Viruses are important pathogens in upper respiratory tract infections. Examples include parainfluenza, influenza, reo, adeno, measles and echo viruses. Important bacterial pathogens in this region are haemophilus, bordetella, *Streptococcus pyogenes*. A major problem associated with viral upper respiratory tract infections and also with bordetella is secondary bacterial infection. Diseases of the lower respiratory tract include lobar and bronchopneumonia. Bacteria are the more important pathogens in this group, e.g. pneumococcus, *Staphylococcus aureus*, *M. tuberculosis*, klebsiella, haemophilus and others. Respiratory syncitial virus, cytomegalovirus and *Pneumocystis carinii*, an organism only pathogenic in the immunosuppressed patient, also cause lower respiratory tract infections. Q fever, psittacosis, *Mycoplasma pneumoniae* are all less common respiratory pathogens. Certain systemic diseases may be acquired by inhalation, e.g. smallpox, measles, mumps, whooping-cough, diphtheria, meningococcal meningitis and/or septicaemia and streptococcal disease.

Diagnosis of respiratory infections depends on history and examination. Special investigations include X-ray examination and the submission of specimens for microbiological examination. Specimens should reach the laboratory as soon as possible. Swabs are submitted from the upper respiratory tract, sputa from the lower respiratory tract. Faeces are also submitted. Viruses are usually present during the first few days of the clinical syndrome — specimens submitted at this time only rarely yield viral growth. The isolation of bacteria is more successful. Problems associated with the interpretation of isolates from specimens from the respiratory tract are appreciable because:

  (i) The specimen is 'contaminated' by normal flora.

  (ii) Certain members of the normal flora are potential pathogens.

  (iii) Antibiotics or a change in the environmental flora, e.g. hospitalization, can lead to alterations in the patient's respiratory flora. Hospitalized patients tend to acquire gram negative bacilli in the oropharynx; antibiotics may encourage the growth of oral candida.

SUMMARY

The respiratory system is:

  (*a*) A portal of entry for micro-organisms.

  (*b*) A site from which dissemination of organisms can occur — patient to patient; staff to patient; patient to staff; staff to staff.

  (*c*) Viruses are responsible for the majority of upper respiratory tract infections, bacteria for the majority of the lower respiratory tract infections.

  (*d*) Diagnosis of the clinical condition is made according to the anatomical site of the lesion; identification of the causative organism is made in the laboratory. *Bordetella pertussis* and adenovirus both cause a clinical 'whoop'. Croup can be caused by *Haemophilus influenzae* and also by the parainfluenza viruses.

  (*e*) Man, by indulging in cigarettes and permitting air pollution, is interfering with the normal defences of his respiratory system.

  (*f*) Sputum is at best a contaminated specimen. The individual collecting sputa is urged to submit a deep cough specimen and not saliva.

Table XXX
VIRUSES RESPONSIBLE FOR THE COMMON COLD

Coxsackievirus   Rhinovirus   Coronavirus   Reovirus   Adenovirus
Influenza   Parainfluenza   Respiratory syncitial

THE URINARY TRACT

The kidney filters the blood removing certain products of metabolism and correcting the body's acid base balance. The renal filtrate flows down the renal pelvis and ureters, emptying into a reservoir. Urine is stored in the bladder and when convenient the bladder is emptied via the urethra. Contraction of the bladder is necessary for the expulsion of urine. During pregnancy and in certain cases of abnormal vesico-ureteric anatomy, urine may reflux up to the ureters during bladder contraction. Vesico-ureteric reflux is a potentially dangerous situation.

The urinary tract is a sterile system. Streptococci, corynebacteria, bacilli and yeasts are all found in the distal urethra. Except for the distal portion of the urethra, no bacteria are normally found in the urinary tract. Urine is a suitable culture media for many bacteria. It is deficient in humoral and cellular defences. The hyperosmolarity of urine inhibits phygocytic activity and decreases the bactericidal effect of serum. Fresh urine, with additional nutrients, is continuously added to the bladder; bladder drainage is intermittent. Bacterial metabolites are diluted and removed at regular intervals. Bacterial multiplication is limited by the acidity of urine. A urea concentration of 2-4% has been shown to be bactericidal. The movement of urine out of the urethra acts as a lavage washing bacteria from the distal urethra.

The male has been shown to be less susceptible to urinary tract infection than the female. This may be due to the following —
(*a*) The presence of bactericidal substances in the prostatic fluid.
(*b*) The length of the urethra. The male urethra is longer than the female.

Bacteria are thought to reach the kidney by one of the following routes:
(i) Bacteria may ascend from the urethra, bladder and ureters. This is an ascending infection.
(ii) Bacteria may spread to the kidney by the blood stream or in the lymphatics.

The major route of kidney infection is due to ascending infection. The danger inherent in vesico-ureteric reflux is apparent.

Urinary tract infection is expressed as bladder infection — frequency, urgency, burning. Kidney involvement is demonstrated by the presence of loin tenderness.

Cystisis is potentially dangerous as the urine reservoir now contains an infective medium. Reflux of urine is now reflux of an infected medium. Acute and later chronic pyelonephritis can lead to renal failure. The relationship between bacteriuria and pyelonephritis, although strongly suspected, is not completely proven.

Factors which are associated with an increased incidence of urinary tract infection are:
(i) Anatomical abnormalities of the urinary tract.
(ii) The female sex. Females, possibly due to their short urethras and their sex hormones, are more prone to urinary tract infection than males. Trauma to the urethra during coitus aggrevates this situation.
(iii) Pregnancy is associated with bacteriurea. The urine excreted by the pregnant female is rich in glucose — glucose provides a good substrate for bacterial growth. The pregnant lady is further a victim of her hormonal balance as vesico-ureteric reflux is a common problem during pregnancy.

(iv) The urine of the diabetic patient is a good culture medium.

Infection of the urinary tract can be exogenous or endogenous. Endogenous infection is usually due to bacteria normally found in the patient's bowel, e.g. *E. coli, Strept. faecalis.* Over 70% of community acquired urinary tract infections are due to *E. coli.* It is important to identify the bacterium responsible for an infection. Re-infection with a new organism is about twice as common as relapse due to inadequate or incorrect treatment of the original infection. The bacteria most commonly incriminated in urinary tract infections acquired at home are *E. coli* and *Proteus mirabilis.* In hospitals the incidence of klebsiella, proteus (all four species), pseudomonas and antibiotic resistant *E. coli* is markedly increased. Proteus is especially well adapted to cause infection of the urinary tract. This organism produces urease which splits urea and releases ammonia. The ammonia not only neutralises the acid urine producing a more favourable culture medium, it also inactivates any complement which may be present in the urine. Proteus may also, due to its ability to alkalinize urine, precipitate calculus formation.

In hospitals urinary tract infections are characterized by two features:

(*a*) Infection with antibiotic resistant organisms.

(*b*) Instrumentation of the urinary tract.

Catheterization of females is routinely performed by the nursing staff. The female patient, already at risk with her short urethra, now has a foreign object introduced into her bladder. Absolute sterility must be observed when a patient is being catherterized. Not only must the catheter be sterile but adequate cleaning of the vulvo-vaginal area is necessary. Catheterization and the presence of an indwelling catheter are a major hazard to the hospitalised patient. Organisms may be introduced into the bladder from both the distal portion of the urethra and from the vulvo-vaginal area. Organisms can penetrate the catheter or be introduced between the urethra and catheter tubing. Nursing staff should not manipulate the connection between catheter and urine bag; if manipulation is necessary it should be done with washed hands. Fluid flows downhill, when catheterized patients are turned the urine in the urine bag should not be emptied into the patient's bladder. This can be avoided by keeping the urine bag below the level of the bladder or by clamping off, or draining, the urine bag prior to turning sick patients. Similar precautions should be observed when working with urine bags as are observed when working with underwater intercostal drains.

Indwelling catheters which are complicated by bacteriuria may be managed by bladder irrigation. In the absence of systemic disease, pyrexia, or toxaemia, antibiotics are not routinely given to catheterized patients with a bacteriuria. Antibiotic therapy in these cases is seldom successful before the catheter is removed.

Urinary catheters are a potent source of infection because:

(i) They upset the normal physiology of the area.

(ii) They pass from an unsterile environment into a sterile area.

It is of the utmost importance that:
  (i) Strict aseptic technique is observed during catheterization of a patient.
  (ii) The catheter is removed as soon as the patient's condition permits.

The collection of urine for bacteriological examination is an important procedure which, if incorrectly performed, results in a valueless laboratory report. A mid-stream specimen of urine is collected. A clean catch is attempted. Urine is collected in a sterile container and submitted to the laboratory as soon as possible. Urine is a good culture medium and specimens reaching the laboratory after a delay are of limited value. When a delay of more than one hour between urine collection and submission to the laboratory is anticipated, the urine should be refrigerated. A temperature of 4°C is not conducive to bacterial multiplication. Bacterial multiplication in the urine specimen renders results of little value as the significance of any bacteria found in a urine specimen is determined by the number of organisms present. Occasionally suprapubic puncture is performed to collect a technically sterile urine specimen. If a patient is already catheterized for medical reasons the collection of uncontaminated urine is not a problem.

Salmonella typhi, rubella and cytomegalovirus are excreted in the urine during systemic disease. Urine is therefore a mode of spread for these organisms. An individual with leptospirosis excretes large numbers of organisms in his urine; an individual with bilharzia may excrete viable *Schistosoma haematobium* ova in his urine. This latter urine passed into a snail infested stream converts a safe swimming area into a bilharzial risk. Urine may therefore act as a vector of disease.

Urine is reputed to kill hookworm ova!

SUMMARY
  (i) Urine is a normally sterile fluid. The presence of organisms in correctly collected urine implies cystitis or urinary tract infection. Occasionally organisms responsible for systemic disease are excreted in the urine.
  (ii) Bladder instrumentation is a major factor in the incidence of hospital acquired urinary tract infections. Catheterization assumes rating as a hazardous procedure in view of the risk of introducing bacteria into the urinary tract.

THE GENITAL TRACT

The female genital tract is subject to alterations in pH and thus resistance to certain infections varies at various stages of a woman's life. The hormones initiating and maintaining the menstrual cycle are also responsible for production and storage of glycogen in the vaginal cells. Lactobacilli

are normal vaginal commensals and these organisms metabolise the glycogen, converting it into lactic acid. The vaginal pH is therefore acid as
long as the hormones stimulating glycogen are present. The pre-pubertal
and post-menopausal female lacks this protective mechanism. Other members of the normal vaginal flora include clostridia, peptostreptococci and
β-haemolytic streptococci group B.

The transfer of normal vaginal commensals into other anatomical sites
can present a problem. Group B streptococci can be aspirated by the baby
during its passage through the birth canal. The premature infant is particularly at risk of fatal meningitis and/or septicaemia as a result of group B
infection. Clostridia are a potential hazard to a person requiring an above
knee amputation for peripheral vascular disease.

Vaginal infections are often associated with one or more of the following:

(i) the menopause;

(ii) local antibiotic pessaries;

(iii) diabetes.

Vaginal candidiasis is a common complaint. The white plaques characteristic of candida infection are found in the vaginal mucosa. *Trichomonas
vaginalis* grows well in a neutral pH and causes a frothy irritating vaginal
discharge. This organism is venereally transmitted. Asymptomatic infection of the male prostate can result in repeated reinfection of the female
partner. Treatment of both partners is therefore essential.

Certain vaginal or genital infections are more related to sexual exposure
than to the vaginal defence mechanisms. The venereal diseases require
intimate contact in order for the organism to be spread from one individual to the next. These organisms succumb to drying, heat, cold and other
environmental conditions.

Table XXXI
A LIST OF VENEREAL DISEASES

DISEASE	ORGANISM
Non-gonococcal urethritis	Chlamydia group or other agents suspected
Gonorrhoea	*Neisseria gonorrhoeae*
Syphilis	*Treponema pallidum*
Chancroid/Soft sore	*Haemophilus ducreyi*
Lymphogranuloma venereum	Chlamydia group B
Lymphogranuloma inguinale	*Donovania granulomatis* (organism related to klebsiella)

Gonorrhoea is clinically characterized by dysuria in the male. A percentage of females are asymptomatic. Infection of the genital mucosa by
gonococci requires that the organism adhere to the mucosal cells by pili.
The pili confer on the organism the ability to resist phagocytosis and also
the ability to cling and remain attached to the mucosa in the presence of

the urine stream. About 10% of males with gonorrhoea are asymptomatic; a very much higher percentage of females are asymptomatic carriers.

Non-gonococcal urethritis, like gonorrhoea, presents as dysuria. Many of the other venereal diseases present with a local lesion on the genitalia, e.g. syphilis, chancroid.

Table XXXII

VENEREAL DISEASES WITH A LOCAL LESION

DISEASE	LOCAL LESION	DRAINING LYMPHADENOPATHY
Primary syphilis	Indurated chancre	Hard and non-tender
Chancroid	Ulcer	Tender
Granuloma inguinale	Granulomatous lesion	May discharge pus
Lymphogranuloma venereum	Vesicles and papules	Adenitis leads to fibrosis

The venereal diseases responsible for systemic disease are syphilis and less frequently gonorrhoea.

Other diseases transmitted by sexual intercourse are herpes group II and the virus responsible for serum hepatitis (hepatitis B). Herpes genitalis results in painful vesicles and ulcers on the genitalia — males find intercourse painful and females are particularly prone to relapses at a certain stage of their menstrual cycle. When hepatitis B is transmitted the acute disease may be subclinical.

Table XXXIII

ORGANISMS WHICH MAY BE SPREAD BY SEXUAL CONTACT

ORGANISM	LESION IN THE MALE	LESION IN THE FEMALE
Trichomonas vaginalis	often asymptomatic	vulvo-vaginitis
Candida albicans	often asymptomatic	vulvo-vaginitis, cervicitis
Herpes II	painful blisters	painful blisters
Neisseria gonorrhoea	urethritis	often asymptomatic
Treponema pallidum	painless chancre	chancre often not observed
Haemophilus ducreyi	suppurating ulcer	ulcer
Chlamydia (Lympho-granuloma-venereum)	painless vesicles	lesion missed in early stages
Chlamydial urethritis	urethritis	asymptomatic
T-mycoplasma (?non-gonococcal urethritis)		

Venereal disease is on the increase. Certain sources rate the annual world gonorrhoea incidence at one hundred million cases. In certain geographical areas non-gonococcal urethritis is more prevalent than gonorrhoea. The increase in the incidence of venereal disease is attributed to a number of different factors.

(i) Social causes —

  (a) Industrialization and centralization concentrating the population in large cities.
  (b) An increase in leisure time.
  (c) An alteration in the social norms.
  (d) Loss of the fear of pregnancy due to 'safer' contraception.
  (e) Less use of the condom.

(ii) Medical factors —

  (a) The increased resistance of gonococci to penicillin.
  (b) Improved diagnostic techniques.
  (c) Better contact tracing.

SUMMARY

(1) A number of different groups of organisms may be transmitted venereally — amongst the viruses — herpes II and hepatitis B; amongst the bacteria — *T. pallidum, N. gonorrhoea, H. ducreyi;* amongst the protozoa — *Trichomonas vaginalis;* amongst fungi — *C. albicans;* and chlamydia. T-mycoplasma are suspected genital pathogens.

(2) The incidence of venereal disease is proportional to the sexual exposure and promiscuity of the individual and the population.

(3) The female genital tract enjoys a better superficial defence barrier during the reproductive years of a woman's life than before this period.

(4) Certain venereal diseases may be diagnosed in one partner while the other partner is an asymptomatic carrier. In the control of venereal diseases it is necessary to treat both partners.

THE SKIN

The skin is one of the well recognised components of man's superficial defence barrier. It boasts mechanical, chemical and microbial components. The mechanical aspect of this barrier is subject to breaches in the hospital environment due to the surgeon's knife, the intern's intravenous drip and the nurse's injection needle. The microbial barrier consists of organisms well adapted to skin conditions. Micro-organisms establishing themselves on skin are subject to shedding as the superficial squamous epithelial cells desquamate. The skin is also often too dry for the prolonged survival of pathogens. Constant contact between the skin and the environment leads to two different bacterial population groups —

  (a) The resident flora: These are organisms which are well adapted to skin conditions and are consistently isolated from the skin. Examples of resident bacteria include staphylococci, corynebacteria. Non-pathogenic mycobacteria are found in areas rich in sebaceous glands; fungi, e.g. yeasts, are found in skin folds where conditions are moister.

(*b*) Transitory flora: These organisms are subject to changes. They may be carried for only a limited period of time.

Neither washing nor scrubbing significantly alters the resident flora of the skin. Hexachlorophene, an antiseptic agent against gram positive cocci, is used by theatre staff in an effort to decrease the gram positive organisms on their hands and forearms. Regular frequent use of hexachlorophene leads to a residual anti-bacterial effect due to penetration of this agent into the glands of the skin. A single application has no significant or prolonged effect on resident flora.

The chemical skin barrier is associated with an acid pH, the presence of toxic fatty acids in sebaceous secretions and the saline and lysosomal content of sweat. Sweat is the secretion of eccrine glands.

Breaches in the skin can lead to local skin infections or to systemic disease. Systemic disease may also be associated with skin manifestations in the form of skin rashes. Numerous members of both the kingdoms of the Protista and Arthropoda are responsible for skin lesions. Only certain important skin diseases will be mentioned.

VIRAL CAUSES OF SKIN LESIONS

Viruses cause a number of different skin lesions. Four basic types can, however, be differentiated.

(*a*) The macular-papular skin lesion. Different degrees of these two basic components may be found in rashes caused by, e.g. rubella, rubeola and enteroviruses.

(*b*) A vesicular rash. Vesicular rashes may in the early phases be macular and may, after the formation of vesicles, progress further to pustules or scabbed areas. The depth of the skin lesion will determine if residual scarring will result. Two viral groups causing vesicular rashes are the poxviruses including smallpox, and the herpes viruses including chicken-pox.

(*c*) Haemorrhagic rashes. Any of the above rashes may develop a harmorrhagic component. In certain cases the haemorrhage into the skin is a result of platelet insufficiency. Certain members of the arbovirus group are recognised as agents causing haemorrhagic rashes. Haemorrhagic measles is a well recognised entity.

(*d*) Skin tumours. *Molluscum contagiosum* and the human wart virus are both DNA viruses which cause skin tumours or warts.

RICKETTSIA AND SKIN LESIONS

Rickettsial diseases give rise to a macular-papular skin rash. The nobbly papular component of the rash is marked.

BACTERIAL CAUSES OF SKIN LESIONS

Bacteria can give rise to different skin lesions, e.g. secondary syphilis is manifest by a maculo-papular rash, meningococcaemia is accompanied by a macular skin rash which may become haemorrhagic. A chronic skin ulcer may be due to *Mycobacterium ulcerans* or *Mycobacterium marinum*.

Tuberculosis, a systemic disease, can occasionally seed organisms to the skin. Leprosy is a disease that has skin and peripheral nerves as its target organ. In hospital there are two organisms that are of especial significance in skin infections. These are *Streptococcus pyogenes* and *Staphylococcus aureus*. Both of these organisms are a particular danger in surgical and neonatal units. Staff with streptococcal or staphylococcal skin lesions should be excluded from these areas. Streptococci, and more especially staphylococci, are carried by a number of healthy individuals in their upper respiratory tract. Nasal staphylococcal carriers present a particular problem. The wearing of masks is an attempt to decrease this problem.

Lesions caused by *Streptococcus pyogenes* include:

(i) Impetigo — a highly infectious skin condition. The superficial layers of the skin are infected and form golden crusts.

(ii) Ecthyma — a deeper lesion with a thicker crust which leaves residual scarring.

(iii) Erysipelas — the organism commonly invades the skin through invisible breaches, but surgical wounds may also become infected. Erythema and swelling are typical.

(iv) Cellulitis — a spreading skin lesion.

(v) Scarlet fever — this is a skin manifestation of a systemic infection by the organism. *Streptococcus pyogenes*, when infected by a particular bacteriophage, develops the ability to secrete erythrogenic toxin. This toxin is responsible for the rash in scarlet fever.

(vi) Sensitization or allergic lesions — in certain diseases caused by *Streptococcus pyogenes*, skin rashes may reflect overtones of the imbalance between host and parasite, e.g. in rheumatic fever the host may develop erythema marginatum or erythema nodosum.

Skin infection by *Streptococcus pyogenes* can be the factor initiating acute glomerulonephritis in certain individuals.

Staphylococcus aureus is possibly the single most important organism in certain hospital wards. The clinical manifestations of the disease depend on the site of the organism, e.g. invasion alongside of a hair follicle gives rise to a localized folliculitis; subcutaneous convergence of several adjacent infected hair follicles cause a carbuncle. An abscess starts in many cases as a staphylococcal infection. Staphylococci can cause different forms of impetigo. In infants and young children bullous impetigo can lead to systemic disease and death. This form of impetigo is highly contagious. An important reason for the obligatory gowning, gloving and masking of persons entering neonatal nurseries is staphylococcal bullous impetigo. In adults staphylococcal impetigo is a benign pustular crusted lesion. A particular *Staph. aureus* is capable of causing the scalded skin syndrome (toxic epidermal necrolysis) in the young. The neonate and young infant are particularly susceptible to infection by this organism. A toxin is secreted by the organism which acts on the skin at the level of the stratum granulosum, resulting in skin peeling.

Staphylococcal septicaemia can also give rise to skin lesions. These lesions are generally haemorrhagic with necrotic areas.

The introduction of an epidemic strain of staphylococci into a neonatal ward results in rapid colonization of 90% of the infants. Some of these infants will develop overt disease while others will become asymptomatic carriers. They may transmit the organism to newborn babies joining them in the unit; they may also infect their mothers, giving them mastitis and a breast abscess. The staphylococcus is just as great a problem in the surgical ward. Surgical wounds with their sutures provide an excellent site for staphylococcal infection. The infective dose of staphylococci is decreased by 1 000 to 10 000 times in the presence of foreign material — including suture material.

Certain other bacteria may colonize wounds. Pseudomonas is a particular hazard in burns patients, while *Clostridium perfringens* is a danger in anaerobic necrotic skin lesions.

SKIN LESIONS DUE TO FUNGI

Ringworm or dermatophytosis is an important superficial fungal infection of the skin. Candida is particularly common in moist skin fold areas. Candida causes paronychia as frequently as staphylococci.

Many other fungi cause skin lesions. These are less commonly encountered and include sporotrichosis, mycetoma and chromomycosis, a warty lesion. Certain systemic fungal diseases may invade the host using the skin as a portal of entry.

SUMMARY

(1) The skin is one of the natural superficial barriers of defence.

(2) The skin may be the target organ in certain local infections, e.g. cellulitis; it may act as the portal of entry for certain systemic diseases, e.g. tetanus, and it may be one of the organs experiencing changes due to systemic infections, e.g. jaundice due to viral hepatitis.

(3) Infective skin lesions may participate in the spread of disease by direct contact or by shedding of bacteria into the environment.

(4) Many different micro-organisms are capable of infecting the skin. The most important of these in the hospital situation is *Staphylococcus aureus*.

(5) The skin has a limited range of reactions available to it — it may form a macule (an area of redness), a papule (a raised area), a vesicle (a blister) or a pustule (a vesicle with pus). Haemorrhage may occur into any of these lesions. Skin death leads to an ulcer or necrotic area. Deeper lesions of the skin can lead to brawny induration or abscess formation. Occasionally the skin can produce warty masses in response to infection.

THE CARDIO-VASCULAR SYSTEM

The cardio-vascular system represents one of the normally sterile anatomical areas. Invasion of the blood stream by bacteria may occur from breaches in the skin, or mucous membranes. Infection of any organ system may be associated with a bacteraemia, e.g. pneumococcal pneumonia can often be diagnosed by the presence of lung pathology and a positive blood culture. Certain diseases are typically characterized by the blood spread of organisms during particular phases of the illness, e.g. typhoid, measles. During mastication or any dental manipulation, commensal oral bacteria may, for a short period, be found in the blood stream.

In hospitals, intravenous and/or intra arterial catheters are a potential source for the introduction of bacteria or fungi. Removal of these catheters is often followed by the conversion of a hitherto positive blood culture to negative.

The presence of bacteria in the blood stream can result in two different types of complications:

(*a*) The bacteria can multiply. Bacterial products may be released and severe patient reactions may occur, e.g. endotoxic shock. These organisms may settle in previously normal organs, e.g. a staphylococcal abscess in the kidney. Septicaemia may develop in a previously healthy individual.

(*b*) The second syndrome of complications associated with release of bacteria into the blood stream is related to a select group of patients. Patients who have previously suffered damage to their heart valves, be it due to rheumatic fever, arthrosclerosis and calcification, or cardiac surgery, are at risk of developing subacute bacterial endocarditis. The organisms settle and multiply in vegetations (clots) which have formed on the damaged heart valves. These organisms are then shed into the blood stream at intervals. The organisms can cause further damage to the heart valve. The patient may develop congestive cardiac failure or may suddenly demise due to rupture of the valve.

Organisms commonly implicated in subacute bacterial endocarditis are *Streptococcus viridans* and *Streptococcus faecalis*. In hospital practice Gram-negative organisms are today more commonly cited as agents causing bacteraemia than Gram-positive cocci.

When specimens are being collected for blood culture, extreme care must be taken in order to avoid contamination of the specimen. Contamination of the specimen by a single skin bacterium can lead to diagnostic and therapeutic headaches.

SUMMARY

(1) Introduction of invasive bacteria into the blood stream may result in septicaemia. Gram-negative bacilli are the group of bacteria most frequently implicated in nosocomial septicaemia.

(2) Patients who have damaged heart valves are at risk of developing infection of these rough surfaces.

(3) The danger of endocarditis is increased in hospitals where invasive procedures may precipitate a bacteraemia. These procedures include prostatic examination, sigmoidoscopy and vascular catheterization.

THE GASTRO-INTESTINAL TRACT

The gastro-intestinal tract (GIT) is that organ system responsible for digestion and absorption of nutrients. The food which enters the GIT enters a tube with an orifice at both ends. During its passage through this tube food is subject to the effects of digestive enzymes acting in the stomach at an acid pH, and in the duodenum at an alkaline pH. The duration of contact between digested food and the absorptive surface of the mucosa is determined by gut motility. Absorption is a function of the stage of digestion which food has reached, the food mucosal contact time and the presence of normal mucosa. Dysfunction of this organ system can be expressed by a change in motility — increased motility results in diarrhoea, decreased motility in constipation. Malabsorption of food may result in weight loss, anaemia, steatorrhoea and general ill health.

With each mouthful of food ingested micro-organisms are introduced into the gastro-intestinal tract. The bacterial count in a fasting stomach is very low — 10-100 organisms per gram of stomach contents. After a meal this count rises to between one million to one hundred million organisms per gram of stomach contents. Half the bulk of faeces is composed of living bacteria or their remains. The superficial barrier of the GIT consists of:

(*a*) A mechanical component — Peristalsis moves intestinal contents, including bacteria, towards the anal orifice.

(*b*) A chemical component — the acid barrier in the stomach kills many micro-organisms. Most of the pathogenic micro-organisms are susceptible to an acid pH of 1-2.

(*c*) A microbial component — faeces consist of bacteria, undigested residual food and various other alimentary secretions and excretions. Faeces may contain as many as 10^{12} organisms per gram. The bacterial count decreases from the large intestine, where a count of 10^{10} organisms per gram of contents is common, to counts of 10^2 or 10^3 organisms per gram of small intestinal contents. It has been shown that the normal intestinal flora has a protective effect.

The normal intestinal flora interferes with superinfection or colonization by pathogenic organisms. The mechanism whereby this protective effect is achieved is not proven but various postulates have been made. The normal bowel flora is well adapted to environmental conditions in the bowel; the pathogens may find the environment created by the digestive processes and the resident bacteria less than ideal. Resident bowel flora are predominantly anaerobic. Bacteroides, the organism present in largest numbers in the bowel, is a strict anaerobe whose growth is stimulated by bile salts. Competition between residents and pathogens for nutrients and space may play an important role. Certain of the residents may produce products toxic to any would-be intruder.

Various humoral secretory products may also play a role in protection of the intestine against infection. Lysozyme has been detected in intestinal secretions — its importance has, however, not been accurately assessed. Secretory IgA is produced by local lymphoid tissue. This antibody is resistant to digestion by the enzymes present in the lumen of the intestine. IgA is capable of activating complement by the indirect pathway. The presence of IgA in the intestinal lumen is thought to play an important role in the resistance of the gastro-intestinal tract to infection. IgA found in faeces is termed coproantibody.

Breast milk provides both maternal antibody and lactoferrin, a bacteristatic compound, to the neonatal GIT.

The intestine can provide a portal of entry for agents causing a wide spectrum of disease patterns:
- (*a*) Organisms causing systemic disease, e.g. typhoid, polio, infectious hepatitis, enter the body by means of ingestion.
- (*b*) Ingested ova hatch in the intestine. The larva may leave the intestinal tract to wander about the body before returning to the intestinal lumen as an adult, e.g. ascaris.
- (*c*) Local infection of the intestinal tract may occur.

The presence of intestinal bacteria can lead to the following clinical syndromes:
- (*a*) Malabsorption.
- (*b*) Dysentery or diarrhoea.
- (*c*) Coma associated with liver failure.
- (*d*) Metabolites of intestinal bacteria have been postulated to bear an aetiological relationship to colonic carcinoma.

BACTERIAL INFECTION OF THE GIT

(*a*) *Malabsorption:* This can occur as a result of the blind loop syndrome leading to excessive localized bacterial proliferation. The equilibrium between bacteria and the small intestine is disrupted, leading to interference with digestion. Digestion may be impaired as a result of competition for nutrients, due to decomposition and deconjugation of bile salts or due to the production of irritant metabolites.

(*b*) *Diarrhoea and dysentery:* Diarrhoea is the frequent passage of unformed stools. Dysentery implies inflammation of the bowel wall and hence the presence of blood, mucus and cells in the stool.

Mechanisms whereby diarrhoea or dysentery may occur:
- (i) Due to enterotoxin secretion — Enterotoxin is an exotoxin secreted by certain intestinal pathogens, e.g. *V. cholerae*, enteropathogenic *E. coli*. Enterotoxin attaches to the mucosal cells of the small intestine causing stimulation of adenyl cyclase activity. Adenyl cyclase

is an enzyme which controls fluid and electrolyte secretion. Increased adenyl cyclase activity leads to a nett outpouring of fluid and electrolytes into the small intestine. Absorption is normal. Enterotoxin acts on the small bowel.

(ii) The bacteria may invade the mucosal cells, resulting in destruction of the superficial epithelial cells, e.g. shigella, invasive *E. coli.*

(iii) The host's immune response to bacteria surviving within phagocytes may be responsible for the diarrhoea in salmonellosis.

Diarrhoea can be a result of intoxication or infection. Intoxication occurs when a preformed toxin is ingested, e.g. as in *Staph. aureus*, and *Clostridium botulinum* food poisoning. Infection is due to the ingestion of viable bacteria. The pathogenesis of this diarrhoea is related to the multiplication of the organisms within the bowel. Examples of organisms causing infective diarrhoeas include *V. cholerae, Salmonella species*. Shigella dysentery is an infection.

The presence of the pathogen in the small intestine often leads to a watery diarrhoea, e.g. *V. cholerae*, toxigenic *E. coli*. The pathogens causing dysentery — a bloody diarrhoea — are usually found in the large intestine.

Bacteria may therefore alter the bowel's motility either by production of extracellular toxins or by invasion of mucosal cells.

(c) *Hepatic coma:* Patients who have suffered severe liver damage as a result of yellow fever, viral hepatitis or toxin ingestion are subject to liver failure and hepatic coma. The liver is no longer capable of adequately playing its role as an organ of detoxification. In cases of liver failure the brain is exposed to toxic substances absorbed from the intestinal tract.

Bowel bacteria produce a variety of metabolites. One of the chief by-products of protein catabolism in the bowel is the conversion of protein and urea to ammonia and various active amines. Ammonia has been particularly incriminated in the pathogenseis of hepatic coma.

Patients with serious liver disease or liver failure therefore have a restricted protein diet and attempts are made to decrease the bowel bacteria by using both antibiotics and purgatives. The presence of blood in the bowel of the patient with liver failure can precipitate hepatic coma.

(d) *Bacteria and colonic carcinoma:* Colon cancer is one of the most important cancers in modern society. Many of the postulated aetiologies involve dietary habits of modern man. The carcinogen(s) responsible for colonic cancer are thought to be produced *in situ*. Bacterial action on intestinal secretions or on dietary constituents has been postulated to produce carcinogenic substances. Bacterial metabolism of sterols and various amino acids, e.g. tryptophan, are suspect. Bacteria may also convert primary amines in the presence of nitrite into carcinogenic nitrosamines. Certain foodstuffs have nitrites incorporated to inhibit the growth of *Clostridium botulinum*. It is feared that these may be converted to nitrosamines by intestinal bacteria. This is the theory behind the uncertainty expressed by certain people about the consumption of red preserved meats.

VIRAL INFECTION OF THE GIT

Certain viruses are regularly found in the gut, e.g. echo and adenoviruses. These may be normal commensals or be associated with disease. Many viruses are suspected of causing diarrhoea — the rotaviruses, a member of the togavirus group, and the parvoviruses, feature prominently on this list.

PROTOZOA AND INTESTINAL DISEASE

Amoebic dysentery is caused by invasion of the large intestine by *Entamoeba histolytica*. Differentiation between amoebic and bacillary dysentery or shigellosis is rapidly achieved by direct examination of the stool at the bedside.

Guardia lamblia and *Balantidium coli* are other protozoan organisms implicated in human disease.

INFESTATIONS OF THE GIT

A number of adult worms can inhabit the intestine of man. Certain of these worms are ingested as eggs, e.g. ascaris, others penetrate the skin, e.g. hookworm. The two species mentioned have a systemic migration and return to live as adults in the small intestine. Other worms are ingested, e.g. enterobius, taenia, and mature in the lumen of the intestine. These worms never penetrate the intestinal mucosa and embark on systemic spread. Taenia is found in the small intestine, enterobius and trichuris in the caecum. Man may ingest these parasites as ova or in their larval forms.

The presence of adult worms in the intestine may be detected by the excretion of eggs in the faeces.

Submission of faecal specimens

Faecal specimens may be collected as portion of stool or in the form of a rectal swab. Collection of specimens for anaerobic organisms must be made under anaerobic conditions.

Control of diseases spread by faecal-oral transmission

Many diseases are spread by the faecal oral route. Organisms may be passed on the faeces of both patients and carriers. The organisms may then directly or indirectly, by soiled hands or fomites, contaminate food and water. In general, diseases are communicable from the end of the incubation period to the onset of convalescence.

Patients suffering from typhoid or cholera should be nursed in semi-isolation. Nursing staff should take particular care in the handling of these patients' excreta. The excreta should be treated prior to disposal, e.g. the rice water stool of the cholera patient may be collected in a bucket containing disinfectant. Nursing staff entering the patient's cubicle should glove and gown. Hand washing on leaving is essential. The patient's eating utensils and bedlinen should be kept separate, and not mixed with that of the general ward.

Nursing of patients excreting pathogenic bacteria is orientated towards breaking the faecal-oral transmission cycle in the patient and preventing the creation of this cycle between the patient and others. Careful handling of excreta and good hygiene are essential.

SUMMARY

(1) Infectious diseases of the GIT are usually acquired by the faecal-oral route. The prevention of these diseases can largely be achieved by the implementation of adequate sanitation and hygiene. Control depends on interrupting the faecal-oral cycle.

(2) A wide spectrum of organisms are capable of being spread by the faecal-oral route and of causing diseases of the GIT, e.g. worms, protozoa, bacteria and viruses.

(3) Some ingested agents cause local disease, others cause systemic disease.

(4) The GIT is endowed with good host defences.

Table XXXIV

DISEASES OF THE GASTRO-INTESTINAL TRACT

VEHICLE	CAUSATIVE ORGANISM
FOOD POISONING	*Clostridium botulinum*
	Staphylococcus aureus
FOOD-BORNE INFECTION	*Salmonella species*
	Brucella species
	Mycobacterium tuberculosis or *M. bovis*
	Bacillus cereus
	Clostridium perfringens
	Rarely Shigella
	Vibrio parahaemolyticus
MILK-BORNE DISEASE	*Salmonella species*
	C. diphtheriae
	Strept. pyogenes
	Brucella
	Mycobacterium bovis
WATER-BORNE DISEASE	*V. cholerae*
	Salmonella typhi
	Leptospirosis
	Hepatitis A
	Poliovirus

THE JAUNDICED PATIENT

Jaundice may result from any insult or disease process in the liver which results in loss of functional hepatocytes. Jaundice is also a feature of a number of different infections. Jaundice due to diseases caused by infective agents includes malaria, yellow fever and leptospirosis. From the hospital viewpoint the most commonly encountered infectious cause of jaundice is that associated with viral hepatitis. Infectious hepatitis is due to hepatitis A virus which is transmitted by the faecal-oral route. When the serum bilirubin reaches its peak or the jaundice is most intense, then the patient is no longer capable of transmitting the virus. The main danger period is before the patient becomes jaundiced and before the diagnosis is made — during this period the patient is excreting the virus and the nursing staff may not be taking adequate precautions. Hepatitis B virus is responsible for serum hepatitis (long incubation hepatitis). This virus is transmitted by injection, especially of blood products, by venereal spread and also occasionally by the oral route. It has also been reported to be secreted in tears. Carriers of hepatitis B may be a hazard to the nursing staff. Hepatitis B presents a particular problem in dialysis units and theatre.

Table XXXV

INFECTIVE CAUSES OF JAUNDICE

VIRAL	BACTERIAL
Hepatitis A virus	Leptospira
Hepatitis B virus	*Treponema pallidum* — congenital
Infectious mononucleosis	*Mycobacterium tuberculosis* — rare
Yellow fever virus	PROTOZOAL
Lassa fever virus	Amoebiasis
Cytomegalovirus — congenital	Plasmodia
Marburg virus	Toxoplasma — congenital
Herpes type I	OTHER
	Chlamydia psittaci
	Coxsiella burnetii

THE SKELETAL SYSTEM

Bones are rigid structures important in providing stability in the human body. They have three anatomical layers — the outer membrane or periosteum, the cortical layer and the inner medulla. Bone infections present a serious problem. Irritation of the periosteum, e.g. in infection, can lead to laying down of new bone and thickening of the cortex. The cortex interferes with drainage of pus and infective material from the medulla. Although the medulla is a blood "lake", the volume of blood supplied to the bone is relatively poor, therefore antibiotics do not generally reach high levels in bone. Poor drainage and inadequate concentrations of antibiotics make bone infections difficult to treat.

Acute infection of bone is called osteomyelitis. Osteomyelitis can result from blood spread or be secondary to trauma, e.g. a compound fracture. *Staphylococcus aureus* is a major culprit. Gram-negative bacilli, e.g. klebsiella, proteus and others are less common but may present problems in orthopaedic units. Children are particularly susceptible to bone infections. The common causative agents of osteomyelitis in this age group are gram positive cocci. Skeletal tuberculosis is usually secondary to tuberculosis elsewhere. Skeletal tuberculosis is characterized by a cold abscess.

Osteomyelitis is an abscess within a rigid cavity and is difficult to cure. Orthopaedic surgery is attended with the risk of bone infection. Of all theatres, the theatre used for orthopaedic surgery is the one where sterility

and asceptic techniques are the most emphasised. All too frequently osteomyelitis requires prolonged antibiotic therapy, surgical drainage and bone
curettage.

Other infections which can result in bone changes include —

(a) *Taenia echinococcus* — cysts of the larval stage of this worm are
commonly found in the liver but may also be found in bone.

(b) Fungal infections of the bone occur. The fungal disease most frequently incriminated is coccidiomycosis.

(c) Leprosy, syphilis and granuloma inguinale all cause bone changes.

(d) Certain viruses can affect bone, e.g. characteristic changes in the
bones of neonates with congenital rubella are found.

The skeletal system consists not only of bones but also of joints. Infection of joints can be due to direct involvement of the joint by an organism.
A joint lesion may also be the result of the host's reaction to the presence
of an organism. Staphylococci can cause acute suppurative arthritis,
Streptococcus pyogenes may cause an immune type of flitting joint pain.
Other organisms recognised to have an aetiological relationship to arthritis
include *N. gonorrhoeae*, brucella, *Mycobacterium tuberculosis* and treponema.

THE CENTRAL NERVOUS SYSTEM

Infection of the brain causes encephalitis, infection of the membrane lining
the brain causes meningitis.

THE BRAIN

Infection of the brain is most commonly due to viruses. Viral encephalitis
may be the presenting system of certain viral infections or it may present
as a complication of a systemic viral disease, e.g. measles, mumps, herpes
type I, infectious hepatitis, smallpox, etc. Echoviruses and certain arboviruses have the brain as their target organ.

The brain is separated from the rest of the body anatomically by the
meninges and the bony cranium. Physiologically it is distinct from all
other organs due to the presence of the blood-brain barrier. This barrier
acts as a protective mechanism whereby substances are selectively transported to, or excluded from, the brain. Any organism reaching the brain
in the blood stream must cross this barrier. The phagocytic cells of the
central nervous system are the microglia.

Encephalitis is clinically manifest as a disturbance of cerebral function.
Signs of infection, e.g. pyrexia, may also be present. Pathologically there
are three different forms of infective encephalitis. Measles may give rise to
any of these forms:

(a) Acute viral encephalitis — This is as a result of viraemia, involving
spread to the brain. The signs of encephalitis occur concurrently
with other signs of the disease, e.g. skin rash. In mumps about half
the cases have a mild form of acute mumps encephalitis.

(b)　Post-infectious encephalitis — This is preceded by the clinical signs of the disease, e.g. the morbilleform rash is present 2-3 weeks before the onset of encephalitis. This form of encephalitis is associated with damage to neurones or their myelin sheath, resulting in the release of encephalitogenic protein. This latter substance is antigenic and induces host antibodies. These antibodies react with the host's neurones. The host is therefore attempting to reject this own brain. The prognosis is poor.

(c)　Subacute sclerosing panencephalitis — Approximately one in every million people who have had measles develop subacute sclerosing panencephalitis. The measles virus genome or an altered genome persists and multiplies in neurones. This is a slow virus disease. With loss of neurones the individual becomes retarded. Subacute sclerosing panencephalitis usually presents one or two years after the acute attack of measles.

　　There is no cure.

Meningoencephalitis is frequently associated with alimentary viruses, e.g. coxsackie, echo and occasionally poliovirus. Meningoencephalitis is clinically characterized by signs of both cerebral involvement and meningeal irritation. There is no loss of consciousness.

Bacterial infection of the brain usually occurs in the form of an abscess. The organism may reach the brain as a result of blood spread or directly due to a fractured base of skull. Brain abscess may complicate a case of meningitis.

THE MENINGES

The meninges are the membranes lining the brain and spinal cord. This is a normally sterile area. The presence of an organism in this area is synonomous with disease. Organisms may reach this area in the blood stream or they may spread directly from the nasal cavity or sinuses through the cribriform plate or through a fractured skull. Meningitis, an infection of the meninges, can be acute or chronic. Bacteria are frequently the pathogens involved. Different organisms assume greater importance in different age groups.

Bacteria causing acute purulent meningitis in the neonate are usually Gram-negative bacilli, e.g. *E. coli*. Babies are particularly susceptible to Gram-negative infections, as IgM, the immunoglobulin which opsonises these organisms, does not cross the placenta. IgG does cross from the mother into the foetal blood stream. At birth the immune system is not fully mature, and these babies are therefore at greater risk than older children. *Streptococcus agalactiae* may cause fatal meningitis and septicaemia in the neonate. The baby is infected during its passage through the birth canal of a maternal carrier. Meningitis in the neonate may have an unusual presentation; a listless, irritable baby who vomits should be suspect. The baby's temperature may be raised or it my be subnormal. A stiff neck is a late sign of meningitis in the neonate.

Three organisms are commonly implicated as the cause of acute purulent meningitis. These organisms are *N. meningitidis*, *Strept. pneumoniae* and *H. influenzae*.

Neisseria meningitidis is responsible for meningitis epidemics. Various groups of this organism are carried in the throat of many individuals. The carrier rate of *N. meningitidis* increases with overcrowding. *N. meningitidis* causes meningitis in all age groups — often following some temporary derangement of host defences, e.g. after a viral illness. Prophylaxis against meningococcal meningitis is in a state of flux. Nursing staff in contact with a patient diagnosed as suffering from meningococcal meningitis were, in the past, all placed on prophylactic sulphonamide therapy. Today certain types of the organism are resistant to sulphonamides. A modern approach to the handling of meningococcal meningitis contacts is to withhold antibiotics and carefully observe the individual. The opportunity to prove this approach is optimal in hospital staff. When prophylactic antibiotics are given minocycline may be used in combination with rifampicin.

The resistance of the meningococcal population to sulphonamides differs in different geographical areas. It is high in Brazil and on the increase in South Africa.

Streptococcus pneumoniae is frequently the aetiological agent of a meningitis which follows a fractured base of skull, otitis media or pneumonia. Owing to the associated pathology in pneumococcal meningitis, the death rate may be higher than that of meningococcal meningitis.

Haemophilus influenzae causes its peak incidence of meningitis in the age group from 4 to 24 months. Outside of epidemic periods, *H. influenzae* is often quoted as being the major cause of meningitis. *H. influenzae* meningitis is well recognised as being followed by complications, e.g. a subdural effusion.

Clinically meningitis is manifest by a stiff neck and pyrexia. When the cerebral tissue becomes involved, changes in the patient's level of consciousness, mentation and personality occur.

Acute bacterial meningitis is a medical emergency. Nursing staff are obliged to wake up any overworked, slumbering casualty officer if they feel that the new case may be a case of meningitis. Early treatment of meningitis may not only save the individual's life, it may also prevent irreversible deafness and mental retardation.

Mycobacterium tuberculosis and *Cryptococcus neoformans* may also cause meningitis. The cerebro-spinal fluid (CSF) picture in these cases differs from the laboratory picture of acute bacterial meningitis. These organisms cause a less acute, often chronic form of meningitis. Aseptic meningitis is a bad term used to describe meningitis where there is a negative bacterial culture of the CSF. Certain viruses, e.g. echo, coxsackie, are the common aetiological agents of aseptic meningitis.

Diagnosis of the type of meningitis depends on the laboratory finding on examination of the CSF. Identification of the agent causing the meningitis determines the treatment. Adequate early treatment of the case determines the prognosis. Cerebrospinal fluid is obtained by lumbar puncture. A needle is pushed through the skin and guided between the lumbar vertebral spines into the meninges. The fluid bathing the brain and spinal cord is then withdrawn. Strict aseptic technique must be observed. Introduction of an organism on the needle or from the overlying skin can lead to infection of this normally sterile area. The cerebrospinal fluid is examined in the laboratory for:

(a) *The causative organism:* This is done immediately by direct examination. A gram stain is used.

Intracellular Gram-negative diplococci are interpreted as *N. meningitidis*, pleomorphic Gram-negative cocco-bacilli as *H. influenzae* and lanceolate gram positive diplococci as *Strept. pneumoniae*. Less commonly other organisms may be seen. In selected cases a Ziehl-Neelsen stain for acid-fast bacilli or an Indian ink preparation for cryptococci may also be performed.

(b) *A cell count:* In acute bacterial meningitis the polymorphonuclear leucocyte cell count is markedly raised. In fungal, viral or chronic bacterial meningitis, lymphocyte counts are important. The presence of cells in the CSF represents the response of the host to irritation of the meninges.

(c) *CSF chemistry:* In acute bacterial meningitis the protein level in the CSF is increased. This is related to the increased permeability of vessels and the increased movement of protein across inflamed linings. The presence of necrotic cells may add to the protein content of the CSF. The sugar level is decreased — this may reflect an increase in metabolism due to the efforts of the phagocytic cells to control the infection. In viral meningitis the sugar level of the CSF is unaffected.

Treatment is started once microscopy and a chemical analysis have been performed. Culture, final identification and drug sensitivity of the organism may follow within 2 or 3 days.

SUMMARY
(1) Meningitis can be caused by a variety of agents. The agents most commonly incriminated are bacteria. The three bacteria most frequently involved are *N. meningitidis*, *H. influenzae* and *Strept. pneumonia*.
(2) Acute bacterial meningitis is a medical emergency. Early, adequate treatment significantly alters the mortality and morbidity of this condition.
(3) Strict aseptic technique is essential when performing a lumbar puncture. The lumbar puncture is an invasive technique temporarily connecting the external environment with the sterile fluid surrounding the central nervous system.

Table XXXVI

EXAMPLES OF ORGANISMS INFECTING CERTAIN ORGAN SYSTEMS

WOUND INFECTIONS
Staphylococcus aureus
Streptococcus pyogenes
Pseudomonas pyocyanea (N.B.: burns)

CHRONIC SKIN LESION
Mycobacteria — atypical, *M. tuberculosis, M. leprae*
Corynebacterium — *C. diphtheriae, C. ulcerans,*
C. minutissimum
Ringworm

SYSTEMIC DISEASE WITH
Neisseria — *N. gonorrhoea, N. meningitidis*

SKIN INVOLVEMENT
Rickettsia
Viral exanthemata of childhood — measles, rubella,
chicken-pox, roseola infantum
Strept. pyogenes in scarlet fever

MENINGITIS

ACUTE	CHRONIC	NEONATE
N. meningitis	*M. tuberculosis*	Gram negative bacilli — *E. coli*
H. influenzae *Strept. pneumoniae*	*Cryptococcus neoformans*	*Strept. pneumoniae* *Strept. agalactiae*

ENCEPHALITIS
Coxsackie
Echovirus
Arbovirus
Also mumps, measles, herpes III viruses

PNEUMONIA
Strept. pneumoniae
Klebsiella pneumoniae
Staph. aureus
Mycobacterium tuberculosis

URINARY TRACT INFECTION
E. coli
Strept. faecalis
Klebsiella
Proteus

SORE THROAT
Strept. pyogenes
Ebstein Barr virus (infectious mononucleosis)
Adenovirus
Coxsackievirus
C. diphtheriae

OTITIS MEDIA
Strept. pneumoniae
H. influenzae
Strept. pyogenes
A complication of measles

SINUSITIS
Strept. pneumoniae
Strept. pyogenes
H. influenzae

CROUP/LARYNGO-
TRACHEO BRONCHITIS
H. influenzae
Parainfluenza virus
Respiratory syncitial virus
Adenovirus

Table XXXVI (*continued*)

SUPPURATIVE LESION	*Staph. aureus* Anaerobic organisms — Peptococci, Peptostreptococci, Bacteroides, Fusobacterium 'Sterile' pus: Mycobacteria
ENDOCARDITIS	*Strept. viridans* *Strept. faecalis* Staphylococcus Rarely rickettsiae, candida
SEPTICAEMIA	Gram negative bacilli — Pseudomonas, *E. coli*, etc. *Staph. aureus* *N. meningitidis*
OSTEOMYELITIS	*Staph. aureus*
CONJUNCTIVITIS	*N. gonorrhoea* — in the neonate *H. aegypticus* Chlamydia Adenovirus
VENEREALLY TRANS- MITTED DISEASE	Bacterial — *T. pallidum, N. gonorrhoea* Chlamydia — lymphogranuloma venereum Viral — herpes II, hepatitis B Mycoplasma *Trichomonas vaginalis* *Candida albicans*
PERITONITIS	*Strept. pneumoniae* Bacteroides *E. coli* Salmonella

CHAPTER 6

Selected Topics

INFECTION DURING PREGNANCY, LABOUR AND THE PUERPERIUM

The pregnant woman is a woman at risk of certain infections. Not only is the expectant mother more susceptible to certain infections, she is also at risk of acquiring infections which may cause harm to her unborn baby.

The foetus develops in a sterile environment. There are, however, two possible routes whereby organisms may reach the unborn child:

(*a*) Via the placenta — the organism may circulate in the maternal blood, e.g. a viraemia or bacteraemia. Transfer across the placenta from maternal to foetal circulation is possible.

(*b*) By an ascending infection of the female genital tract. The organism is postulated to cause an amnionitis prior to infecting the foetus.

As a general principle, the earlier in pregnancy the infection occurs the worse will be the foetal consequences. The first trimester of pregnancy is the period of foetal organogenesis. Infection at this stage can lead to:

(i) Abortion.

(ii) Congenital abnormalities — these are often severe and fatal.

The second and third trimesters are periods of growth and maturation. Infection during this period can lead to:

(*a*) Stillbirth.

(*b*) Congenital abnormalities which may be severe but are more usually compatible with a useful life.

Table XXXVII

FOETAL DEVELOPMENT

Time	Stage of Development
0-6 days —	implantation
6 days-12 weeks —	organogenesis (critical danger period)
12 weeks-term (40 weeks) —	maturation, growth, functional development

Infections leading to congenital abnormalities:

(*a*) Those acquired as a result of transplacental spread —

(i) Congenital rubella ⎱ These organisms cause
(ii) Congenital cytomegalovirus ⎰ congenital malformations.
(iii) Congenital toxoplasmosis ⎱ These organisms cause inflam-
(iv) Congenital syphilis ⎰ mation and destruction.

German measles in the first trimester is considered an indication for therapeutic abortion. Gross abnormalities of the ears, eyes, heart and brain of these children are produced by the presence of the virus in their foetal cells. Rubella infection during the second trimester of pregnancy causes the expanded rubella syndrome. These foetuses are far less severely affected. Deafness remains a problem in congenital rubella infection. Rubella causes lesions in the foetus by slowing down the rate of multiplication of the infected foetal cell. Toxoplasma and cytomegalovirus destroy the foetal cells.

M. tuberculosis and coxsackie B may occasionally be spread transplacentally. Transplacental spread may occur:

    (i) Directly through a healthy placenta, e.g. viral transmission;

    (ii) Through an inflamed placenta, e.g. bacteria; or

    (iii) Through direct vascular connections between maternal and foetal circulation in a placenta with minor vascular anomalies.

  (*b*)   Those acquired by ascending genital infection — ? Herpes group II.

In order for the mother to become infected and spread the organism to her unborn infant during pregnancy, she must not have previously been exposed to, and developed resistance against, the infecting organism.

THE MOTHER

During pregnancy the renal threshold for glucose is lowered and glucose is excreted in the urine. Glucosuria is a consistant finding in the pregnant woman. The uterus and foetus behave as an abdominal mass. All these factors predispose the expectant mother to urinary tract infections. The causative organisms may be *E. coli*, one of the other gram negative bacilli or *Strept. faecalis*.

Vaginal secretions are increased during pregnancy and vaginitis presents a problem.

Immunization and the expectant mother

Immunization of the pregnant female against measles, mumps and rubella is contraindicated. If the expectant mother is travelling to an endemic or epidemic area for yellow fever or polio, she should be immunized against these diseases. Vaccinia can cause disease in the foetus. In the past the risk of infection by the wild strain of variola was greater than that of vaccination. Immune globulin was given at the time of vaccinia inoculation.

Tetanus toxoid is indicated in pregnancy. The immunoglobulins produced by the mother cross the placenta and protect the neonate against tetanus. Immunization against tetanus is especially indicated in certain African tribes where tradition demands the treating of the umbilical cord with cow dung.

INFECTION OF THE NEONATE

The neonatal period is the first 28 days of a baby's life. Included in this section are infections of the baby during its passage down the birth canal.

During the process of birth the baby passes from a sterile environment into a contaminated world teeming with microbes. With the rupture of the membranes, the birth canal is lavaged by the amniotic fluid. The foetus is now in direct contact with a contaminated environment. Prolonged rupture of membranes is associated with an increased incidence of neonatal infections. Prematurity, prolonged labour and instrument delivery are all factors increasing the risk of neonatal infection. During birth the baby may become infected by:

(a) Inhalation of infected material. This is probably the major route of infection.

(b) Direct contact with pathogens, e.g. contact between vaginal discharge and the conjunctiva, or contact between foetal abrasions and maternal faecal soiling.

(c) Ingestion of excretions and secretions.

Once the baby is born, rapid colonization by micro-organisms occurs. The species of micro-organisms to which the baby is exposed is determined by the micro-organisms colonizing the mother, the nursing staff and those present in the environment. The introduction of the neonate to a saphrophytic or pathogenic micro-flora can influence the health of the baby.

Infections acquired during the birth process

Opthalmia neonatorum is infection of the baby's conjunctiva by *N. gonorrhoeae* present in the maternal vagina. Routine instillation of silver nitrate or penicillin eyedrops can prevent blindness in these innocent children.

Streptococcus agalactiae can be inhaled by the baby as he passes down the birth canal. This organism causes meningitis, pneumonia and septicaemia in the neonate. The mortality rate of infected babies in the absence of antibiotic treatment is extremely high.

Herpes II can lead to encephalitis and generalized disease in the neonate. Vaginal candidiasis can lead to oral infections in the newborn.

The neonate

The neonate is at particular risk of acquiring infections caused by Gram-negative organisms. He is also at risk of infection by hospital strains of staphylococci. Maternal IgG antibody is capable of crossing the placenta — IgM does not cross the placenta. Foetal immunity is not fully developed at birth. The foetus is capable of producing antibodies but these are in low concentration and are of a poor quality. The foetus therefore particularly lacks IgM as an antibody defence. IgM is the antibody specialized as an opsonin in the body's early defence against Gram-negative organisms.

Septicaemia, meningitis, diarrhoea, pneumonia and peritonitis are all serious diseases in the new-born. The new-born may react to any of these infections with a paucity of signs. Localizing signs often only develop late in the disease.

Nursery epidemics may be associated with staphylococci, enteropathogenic *E. coli* or coxsackievirus infections. Maternity hospitals may require closure due to outbreaks of coxsackie B myocarditis amongst neonates.

Other organisms important in neonatal infections include listeria, *Strept. faecalis*, pseudomonas, proteus and salmonella.

The neonate at particular risk is:
  (i) premature;
  (ii) delivered after a prolonged labour;
  (iii) traumatised during delivery;
  (iv) delivered hours after rupture of the membranes;
  (v) one with a low Apgar rating;
  (vi) one passing through an infected genital tract.

Nursing home epidemics

(a) The Staphylococcus

Staphylococcus aureus is a normal resident of the skin, anterior nares and throat of 5-30% of individuals. The neonate may thus be exposed to pathogenic cocci carried by its mother, the nursing and medical staff.

Hospital staff are more likely to carry hospital staphylococci than the general population. Hospital staphylococci are selected for by their ability to survive in an environment where antibiotics are used. The typical hospital staphylococcus is one which has developed resistance to antibiotics frequently used in the hospital environment. Hospital staphylococci therefore constitute a greater problem than community acquired staphylococci, as these cocci are likely to demonstrate antibiotic resistance.

Neonatal sites most prone to colonization and infection by organisms are the umbilicus, nose, skin and throat. Diseases caused by staphylococci are usually suppurative, e.g. pustules and furuncles. In the neonate, staphylococcal skin infection may lead to one of two debilitating conditions. Bullous impetigo is characterized by purulent blisters, fever, diarrhoea, bacteraemia and infection of other organs, e.g. the brain, lungs and kidneys. Toxic epidermolysis, also known as the scalded skin syndrome, is related to infection with a specific virulent phage type of *Staph. aureus*. Blistering is followed by scaling of large areas of the neonate's skin. The reaction of neonatal skin to infection may differ from that of the adult. Staphylococcal skin lesions may proceed to septicaemia, meningitis or osteomyelitis. An increasing number of babies with pustules may herald a staphylococcal outbreak in the nursery.

Although hexachlorophene bathing has been shown to decrease the incidence of staphylococcal colonization, it has not definitely been shown to prevent serious disease in neonates. It has, however, been shown to cause brain damage in experimental animals. Hexachlorophene bathing of infants has thus been discontinued in most neonatal units.

The prevention of nursery staphylococcal epidemics is by the exclusion of all staff with staphylococcal infections. Smaller nurseries housing four to six neonates should be used in cycles so that the nursery is cleared between every four to six admissions.

(b) Coxsackie B

These viruses are capable of causing serious disease in neonates. Feeding difficulties and lethargy, with or without fever, in the first eight days of life may be due to coxsackie B infection. Myocarditis or pericarditis may lead to cardiac and respiratory problems. The outcome may be fatal.

Coxsackie B infections are particularly common in children. They cause a wide spectrum of disease — many forms are mild.

It is essential that coxsackie B viruses are not introduced into maternity hospitals. Children are therefore not permitted into maternity units and the number of persons visiting the new mother is strictly limited.

THE PUERPERIUM

The mother who has recently given birth is left with an oozing uterine area where the placenta has detached. Her cervix and perineum may be lacerated. Other factors that increase the mother's susceptibility to infection include:

(a) Early rupture of membranes. Before the membranes rupture about 5% of women have Gram-negative bacilli in their vaginas; by 48 hours after the membranes have ruptured, over 90% of women have Gram-negative organisms colonizing their genitalia.

(b) Prolonged labour, especially if terminated by an instrument delivery is associated with oedema, lacerations and other trauma.

(c) Retained products provide a rich culture medium for organisms. The necrotic material which is retained may further provide anaerobic conditions.

The lower genital tract abounds in a normal flora of anaerobic bacteria. It is also an anatomical area easily soiled by faeces. Problem organisms can include anaerobic organisms, e.g. bacteroides, fusobacterium, clostridia, peptostreptococci. Aerobic organisms are also important, e.g. *E. coli*, staphylococci, *Strept. faecalis*.

Local infection of sutured tears, infection of the inner layer of the uterus (endometritis) and spread to adjacent areas can cause parametritis, salpingitis and peritonitis. In the absence of adequate care and precautions childbirth may be attended by a significant mortality and morbidity.

Breast milk

Mothers may introduce their infants to pathogenic staphylococci; it is, however, usually the infant who introduces a staphylococcus into the maternal breast. A small crack in the nipple, especially in the nipple of an engorged breast, can set the stage for mastitis and breast abscess formation. This apart, mothers feeding their babies on breast milk have several advantages. The milk is manufactured and 'bottled' in a sterile container. The temperature is correct and the concentration of the various constituents supplies, with few exceptions, the infant's dietary requirements.

Breast fed infants tend to have fewer episodes of diarrhoea than bottle fed infants. This may be due to a number of factors, e.g.:

(a) Breast milk contains its constituents in the correct proportions. The infant's gastro-intestinal tract enzymes can adequately digest it.

(b) The milk has not been contaminated during preparation.

(c) Breast milk contains certain anti-microbial factors —

  (i) Antibodies are secreted in colostrum and milk.

  (ii) Unsaturated lactoferrin and transferrin are also secreted. The proteins bind iron. The free iron content of milk is therefore low. Bacteria, e.g. *E. coli*, require iron to stimulate their growth. Enteropathogenic *E. coli* are thought to be an important cause of diarrhoea in infants.

  (iii) Breast milk has a high lactose content. *E. coli* are capable of fermenting lactose and utilizing the energy produced for proliferation. The end product of lactose fermentation is lactic acid production. Human milk has a low protein and low phosphate content and is thus a poor buffer. The lactic acid produced by *E. coli* would lower the pH of the environment and inhibit further growth of the bacterium.

  (iv) The high lactose content encourages the growth of anaerobic lactobacilli which are commensal in the infant's intestine. These organisms create a microbial barrier to pathogens attempting to colonize and infect the intestine. They metabolise lactose to lactic acid and acetic acid, thereby lowering the pH and creating a chemical barrier to pathogens.

  (v) Breast milk contains monocytes. Monocytes are the macrophages of the blood.

ANTIBIOTICS, THE FOETUS AND NEONATE

During pregnancy the expectant mother is prone to infection. Urinary tract infections must be treated as the mother runs the risk of developing pyelonephritis and hypertension. She may also give birth to a dysmature or premature infant. Choice of antibiotic or antimicrobial agent in the treatment of infection in the pregnant female must take into account the sensitivity of the organism and the effect of the drug on the foetus. Once the baby has been born, if the mother is breast feeding, certain drugs may be transmitted to the infant in her milk.

Antimicrobial agents which are avoided in pregnancy due to their effect on the foetus, include streptomycin which may cause deafness and tetracycline which causes abnormal dentition.

Sulphonamides should not be given to the mother after 38 weeks gestation as this anti-microbial agent competes with bilirubin for albumin binding. The foetal liver is deficient in the enzyme necessary to handle bilirubin metabolism. Other drugs which displace bilirubin from albumin include co-trimoxazole, nitrofurantoin and fucidic acid. These agents can all precipitate hyperbilirubinaemia in the neonate.

Drugs that should not be administered to the mother during labour, or to the neonate directly, are:

(i) Chloramphenicol, which can precipitate the Grey baby syndrome with cardiovascular collapse; and

(ii) Nitrofurantoin, which causes haemolysis in this age group.

FEVER

Fever is the most commonly encountered clinical manifestation of inflammation and infection. Fever is not diagnostic of infection. It also occurs in certain neoplastic and collagen diseases. Fever may be induced by drug therapy.

Endogenous pyrogen is the chemical substance responsible for the induction of fever. It is released from a variety of cells, e.g. granulocytes, monocytes and macrophages. Endogenous pyrogen acts on the hypothalamus. The hypothalamus is the centre controlling the preservation and production of heat. In feverish conditions the hypothalamus is normal and healthy but its temperature baseline is pitched at a higher level than usual. In pyrexial patients the blood temperature which triggers the hypothalamus to gear the autonomic nervous system for vasodilation is higher than the acceptable 37,5°C.

Micro-organisms may induce fever in the host by activation of endogenous pyrogen. Phagocytosis of viruses and bacteria by the host phagocytic cells may result in the release of endogenous pyrogen from these cells. Endotoxin, the lipopolysaccharide constituent of gram negative bacterial cell walls, has been clearly shown to induce fever by endogenous pyrogen release. Antibody-antigen complexes also cause release of this pyrogen. Cell mediated immunity results in the release of lymphokines — one or more of these substances is capable of inducing pyrogen activation. Certain micro-organisms are believed to release pyrogenic factors.

Physiologically man reduces his body temperature by vasodilation and sweating. Heat is also lost, especially in animals, by shallow respiration. Salicylates have been shown to decrease the temperature of feverish patients. Salicylates alter the threshold of the hypothalamus and facilitate heat loss.

The value of fever in assisting the host to combat infection remains unknown.

NOSOCOMIAL INFECTIONS

It is naïve to assume that the sole influence of hospitalization on disease is to halt or lessen its progress. A sojourn in hospital is not a passport to health. On the contrary, hospitals constitute an increasingly important source of infections. Hospitals are strongholds of antibiotic resistant bacteria. Many of the organisms, though normally non-pathogenic, are quickly capable of overwhelming the lowered resistance of a sick immunosuppressed patient. Infections acquired in hospital are termed nosocomial infections. Approximately one in every 14 to 17 patients admitted to hospital acquires an infection while in hospital!

The source of the organism may be:

(a) The patients — Individuals may be admitted to hospital suffering from an infection. Patients may be incubating an infectious disease on being admitted for an unrelated complaint. Patients may be carriers of various pathogenic or potentially pathogenic organisms. The latter examples are of special importance. Spread of these organisms can occur in the absence of special precautions.

(b) The staff — Members of the nursing and medical staff are not only good vectors of patient's organisms, they can in addition introduce their own organisms into the hospital. Staphylococci causing minor skin lesions in staff can cause serious wound infection in patients. A mild diarrhoea in a nurse may cause an outbreak of gastroenteritis in the neonatal unit.

(c) The environment — Dust, sinks, flower vases and other fomites are all possible sources of contamination.

Mode of spread: Three main modes of spread occur in hospitals —

(i) Direct contact — This has proved the major mode of spread. The spread of organisms from patient to personnel to patient can be greatly facilitated by poor nursing.

(ii) Indirect contact — Organisms may be spread by inanimate objects, e.g. shigella on door handles, pseudomonas on facecloths. Organisms may also be spread by food.

(iii) Droplet spread — Laminar air flow techniques eliminate this problem. Air conditioners and respirators may aggravate this mode of spread. The obligatory spacing of hospital beds is a practice aimed at lessening the risk of droplet spread between patients.

THE TYPES OF INFECTION

Nosocomial infections may be exogenous or endogenous. Exogenous infections are caused by organisms not normally part of the individual's flora. The organism may be acquired from the nurse, from other patients or from the environment. Endogenous infections are caused by organisms which are carried by the patient himself. Organisms causing endogenous infections may do so by causing infection in a host with a defect in his defences. Organisms normally present in, e.g. the bowel, may cause endogenous infection in an individual by being transferred to a normally sterile site, e.g. the bladder.

Endogenous infections commonly give rise to isolated infections; exogenous infections lead to both sporadic isolated cases and to epidemics.

Two groups of agents are involved in nosocomial infections —

   (i) The pathogens.

  (ii) The opportunists.

Hospital pathogens may be particularly virulent due to a number of factors. An organism which is multiplying and causing active disease in the host may have enhanced virulence. *Yersinia pestis* in the flea lacks fraction I, a major virulence factor. In man with a body temperature of 37°C this virulence factor is produced. Acquisition of *Yersinia pestis* from the bite of a flea is less frequently fatal than acquisition of the organism from a sick individual. Passage of an organism through a number of susceptible hosts has long been recognised as enhancing the virulence of that organism. The pathogen acquired in hospital may thus be particularly aggressive. Hospital pathogens are also subject to selective pressure. Those organisms capable of multiplying in an antibiotic environment are selected for in the hospital environment. Treatment of nosocomial infections may therefore pose a problem. Hospital drug committees suggest changing the antibiotics used in any one ward at regular intervals. This has been shown to decrease the resistant bacterial population to that drug in the unit.

Opportunistic pathogens have an ideal playground in the hospital environment. These organisms which may be commensals or saphrophytes under normal conditions can cause disease when the host's defences are impaired.

In hospital many aspects of the host's defences may be defective.

  (a) *Breaches in the host's superficial defence barrier:* The most common superficial defence barrier to be impaired in hospitals is the skin. Each injection, each intravenous or intra-arterial catheter and each incision made by the surgeon breaches the mechanical defence barrier. Anaesthesia, intubation and urinary catheterization are all procedures interfering with the normal functioning of the superficial defence barrier. Damage to the host's defences may not only be iatrogenic in origin, the patient may enter hospital with burns, abrasions or penetrating wounds.

     Alteration in the host's microbial defence barrier is common in hospital. Patients enter hospital with a 'normal' throat flora. After a few days in hospital they acquire Gram-negative bacilli in their throats. There appears to be a change in colonization immunity in hospital patients.

  (b) *The host's non-specific defences:* The malnourished, the debilitated, the very old, the very young and the sick all have defects in their immune defences.

  (c) *The host's specific defences:* Patients may be on specific immunotherapy. Patients receiving immunosuppression to prevent them rejecting their organ transplant, simultaneously lose the ability to reject micro-organisms. Patients receiving chemotherapy to poison their cancer cells are simultaneously poisoning the cells responsible for specific immunity. Cancer therapy, whether it be by drugs or radio-therapy, is based on the principle that a treatment which is toxic to all living cells will kill the most rapidly multiplying cells first. Both cancer cells and the cells responsible for specific immunity multiply rapidly. Immunosuppressive agents are also used in the treatment of the collagen diseases.

Anatomical zones in particular danger of nosocomial infections depend on the organism, its mode of spread and the defect in the individual patient's defences. Anatomical sites on the danger list are those whose superficial barrier has been impaired, e.g. the urinary tract in the catheterized patient, the lungs in the anaesthetised patient, the skin in the patient with burns or surgical incisions.

Any organism may cause nosocomial infection. The organisms most commonly causing infection in hospitals are bacteria. Staphylococci are of particular importance in surgical and neonatal units. Certain phage types of staphylococci are particularly associated with staphylococcal epidemics. The antibiotic resistance of the hospital staphylococcus is an ever present problem. In the past staphylococci were the major hospital pathogens; today, although these Gram-positive cocci are still important, the Gram-negative bacilli are assuming a major role in nosocomial infections. The increasing incidence of nosocomial infections due to gram negative bacilli is rapidly becoming a major problem. The *Enterobacteriaceae* (*E. coli*, klebsiella, enterobacter) and salmonellae are the chief offenders in this group. Pseudomonas is particularly important in the burns unit.

The spread of respiratory and enteric viruses in hospitals is similar to that in any institution. As therapy for virus diseases is mainly supportive, prevention of these diseases is important. Hepatitis B virus (serum hepatitis) is a serious problem in hospitals. This virus is carried by 5-10% of certain population groups. Spread of hepatitis B virus is in blood and blood products. To avoid spread of this virus in hospitals, hepatitis B positive (dirty) patients and hepatitis B negative (clean) patients requiring haemodialysis, need to be treated on different machines. 'Dirty' patients should ideally be operated upon by hepatitis B positive surgeons and their oozing wounds dressed by hepatitis B positive nurses.

Cytomegalovirus and herpes viruses may cause fatal disease in the immunosuppressed patient. Fungi are also important in patients with a deficient immune response. Candidosis, aspergillosis, cryptococcosis and mucormycosis are all important fungal diseases being encountered with increasing frequency as a consequence of modern medicine.

PRINCIPLES OF CONTROL

The incidence of nosocomial infections is not increasing but it is failing to decrease in the face of greater knowledge and improved techniques. Stricter control and the application of basic principles is recommended. Basic principles include:

(*a*) *Strict surveillance:* A hospital infection team should be created. This team should include medical and nursing personnel. The team should be aware of the admission of patients with infections and the incidence of hospital acquired infections. The incidence of infection in each ward and unit should be recorded. The team should also be aware of the type, frequency and rate of infection associated with invasive procedures in their hospital and in each ward of their hospital. Statistics recording the type of infecting organism, the anatomical site and the incidence of infection of any anatomical site by any single organism should be available. The antibiotics used, the frequency with which they are used, and the resistance of the organisms to these antibiotics should be carefully surveyed and recorded.

By continual surveillance the hospital infection team can detect an increase in antibiotic resistance by any organism in any unit. They can then take steps to decrease this high level of resistance to that antibiotic by restricting use of the drug in that unit. The success of the measures employed by the staff to decrease the level of resistance can be followed by continuing surveillance. A change in the pattern of organisms or the number of infections in a unit may herald the onset of an epidemic. Slackening of aseptic technique in a unit may be detected early and corrected before too much harm is done. The introduction of a particularly virulent organism into the hospital environment can be detected and controlled early.

Adequate continual surveillance can lead to early detection and control of infection. This measure can save lives, decrease morbidity and constitute a significant financial saving for both the individual and the state.

(*b*) *Environmental control:* Biological surveillance of walls, floors, cooking and eating utensils is not generally of much value unless a specific organism is suspected and sought. Regular bacteriological surveys should, however, be carried out on 'sterile' equipment and fluids for intravenous administration.

Hospital design can greatly assist a 'clean' environment. Minimal passage of individuals through any one area, a one way flow of soiled linen and equipment will help to decrease environmental contamination.

(*c*) *Control exercised by the nursing staff:*
(i) Strict aseptic technique: This must extend from the theatre to the dressing of wounds to the catheterization of patients. This technique involves the use of sterile equipment, the prevention of droplet spread by masks and the use of gowns and gloves. It requires the skills necessary in the use of the 'no-touch' technique and the knowledge of how to avoid contamination of sterile equipment and scrubbed hands.
(ii) Nursing staff control an important source of infection in the disposal of the patient's excreta. Shigella, hepatitis B virus and *Vibrio cholerae* are spread in the faeces; urine may contain *Salmonella typhi*, *M. tuberculosis* or even *E. coli*; sputum may be teeming with TB bacilli, pneumonococci, klebsiella or haemophilus. Inadequate

care during disposal of these excreta and the subsequent handling of the container can lead to important breaches in the control of hospital infections.

(iii) Specimens collected in order to be submitted for microbiological examination are suspected by the clinician to contain the organism responsible for the patient's illness. Care during the collection and transport of such a specimen is essential.

(iv) Nursing staff suffering from minor infections may be a source of infection for individuals who are already sick. The nurse with a staphylococcal paronychia can cause wound sepsis or even staphylococcal septicaemia in the theatre case. Members of the nursing staff infected by pathogenic organisms must be excluded from the care of sick patients until their infection is controlled.

(v) It is recommended that only adequately trained staff be employed in high risk areas. A knowledge of sterilization, disinfection and aseptic technique is essential. Undertrained staff, lacking a knowledge of basic microbiology and its application, can unwittingly cause the loss of life.

(*d*) *Hospital procedures associated with a risk of nosocomial infection:* The introduction of foreign material into a patient or the breaching of the patient's superficial defence barrier is fraught with danger. Unless medical and nursing personnel are acquainted with the application of aseptic technique, a diagnostic or therapeutic procedure can initiate a hospital acquired infection.

All wards should have the rule that catheters are removed as soon as possible. Certain wards adhere so strictly to this rule that all intravenous drips are removed at night. Those patients found to still require a drip the following day have a new drip put up early that morning. Urinary catheters should be removed within 48 hours. If no instructions are given regarding the removal of a urinary catheter after 48 hours, the nursing staff may do the patient a favour by inquiring if the catheter is still required. The presence of a urinary catheter is too often associated with the presence of bacteria in the urine to permit any negligence in the care of these patients.

(*e*) *The medical personnel:* These members of the team should:

(i) Limit invasive procedures as far as possible.

(ii) Avoid ward or intensive care unit overcrowding.

(iii) Avoid overburdening the nursing staff — an overworked staff is a less efficient staff.

(iv) Always remember that successful treatment of any underlying disease will boost the patient's general health and therefore his host defences.

(v) Not admit patients for procedures which can safely and efficiently be performed at an outpatient level. Admission of patients for the anti-microbial treatment of a chronic urinary tract infection should be avoided where ethical and possible.

(*f*) *The hospital's antibiotic policy:* Each hospital should have an antibiotic policy. The antibiotic sensitivity of the organisms routinely found in the hospital environment should be monitored. If increasing resistance to a particular antibiotic is noted, then this antibiotic should be withdrawn from use. This procedure has been shown to decrease the resistance of the organism to that antimicrobial agent.

SKIN-BURNS AND WOUND INFECTION

Lesions of the skin constitute an important group of nosocomial infections. Staphylococci present in the hospital dust or in the nose, throat or on the skin of other patients and staff may cause problems in the burns or surgical unit. Organisms infecting burns or wounds arise from the environment, the patient himself, and the hospital staff. Pseudomonas is an organism commonly found in drains and sinks — in the burns patient it may cause a fatal septicaemia.

Arguments rage concerning burn therapy, but a significant proportion of the clinicians treating burns feel that prophylactic anti-microbial therapy is indicated. Topical antibiotics should be avoided.

This concern amongst the clinicians is due to the susceptibility of burnt skin to infection. Impaired circulation is one of the important factors responsible for the susceptibility of burns to infection — a limited number of bacteria may be controlled by a skin surface that has a good blood supply even if the superficial defence barrier has been lost. Infection of a burnt surface by staphylococci, streptococci, pseudomonas or any other organism leads to further skin damage and necrosis. Islets of cells capable of regenerating and reconstituting skin areas are lost due to the damage caused by the infecting organism. Burns may be cleaned and treated by the open or closed method; they may be infected by direct contact, or, if left open, by droplet infection.

The role of the nursing staff in preventing infection of burns starts with admission of the patient into the hospital. In the case of incisions the nurse's role starts before the first surgical incision.

Prior to surgery the patient's skin is prepared, i.e. disinfected using certain antiseptics. The choice of antiseptic used is selected on its ability to destroy the organisms most likely to be present on the skin, i.e. gram positive cocci. Once in the theatre, the patient and the theatre staff are clothed in sterile clothing. The staff involved in the operation are gloved, gowned, masked and wear caps. During the operation care is taken to remove any foreign material from wounds acquired prior to admission. The surgeon's incision is made with a sterile scalpel and care is taken to avoid unnecessary trauma to the tissues. The wound is carefully sutured, care being taken to avoid haematoma formation. The incision is dressed in the theatre.

In the dressing of wounds and burns, strict aseptic precautions must be observed. Dressings should not be performed in the ward but in special dressing rooms. Ideally no nurses carrying staphylococci in their nose or throat should be permitted to dress wounds.

URINARY TRACT INFECTION

The high incidence of urinary tract infections in hospital is partially due to catheterization. Patients may require catheterization for a number of reasons — they may require catheterization for a very limited period or for an extended period, e.g. those who suffer spinal cord lesions. Organisms may be introduced into the bladder during and after the introduction of the catheter.

The distal urethra is a contaminated area through which the catheter passes. The up till now sterile catheter may push these organisms into the bladder. Organisms are also capable of passing between the urethra and catheter. The catheter once inserted may become contaminated by faecal organisms or by handling with unwashed hands. These organisms may then make their way into the bladder along the catheter. Organisms may be transferred by retrograde flow from the urine bag into the bladder. This does not occur spontaneously but requires the assistance of a willing but untrained pair of hands.

The types of organisms responsible for urinary tract infections include *E. coli*, klebsiella, proteus, pseudomonas and enterobacter. These organisms may all be introduced into the bladder by contact and contamination of the catheter system.

The female patient is catheterized by members of the nursing staff. The introduction of a sterile catheter requires application of the 'no-touch' technique by a gloved, gowned and masked individual. Cleansing of the vulvo-vaginal area is essential and must be meticulously performed.

Once a catheter has been introduced, minimal handling of the catheter, the catheter urine bag connection and the urine bag is recommended. The urine bag should be drained rather than changed. Contact with the catheter should only be made with well washed or gloved hands.

Catheters should be removed 48 hours or less after insertion.

BACTERAEMIA

In bacteraemia, the source of the organisms is usually —

(*a*) infection elsewhere in the body, e.g. urogenital tract, skin, respiratory system; or

(*b*) associated with invasive procedures, e.g. intravenous therapy, intra-arterial catheters.

The *Enterobacteriaceae* are the common causative organisms. *Staphylococcus aureus* is also frequently incriminated. When mixed infections occur pseudomonas and fungi are often listed.

Certain sites are prone to infection, e.g. the urinary tract and skin. Nurses can influence the rate of infection in these areas — an effort to limit the number of infections in these areas can lead to a decrease in the incidence of nosocomial bacteraemias.

The nursing staff controls the replacement of empty vacolitres attached to intravenous catheters. The solution being run into the patient's veins often contains dextrose, a good nutrient for bacteria. Care must be taken in breaking the seal of the bottle and connecting the vacolitre with the drip system. Drips must not be allowed to run dry and must regularly be checked for leakage at the skin insertion. Dressings in this area can be soaked in a good bacterial culture media, e.g. plasma. Infection at the site of skin and catheter is a real danger especially in leaky connections. Drips which have run into tissues should be turned off and removed. Damage to tissues leads to decreased local host resistance to infection.

Any tube connecting the patient to the environment is a danger area.

NEONATAL NOSOCOMIAL INFECTIONS

Neonates may acquire organisms from their mothers, members of the hospital staff and other babies. *Staphylococcus aureus*, *Streptococcus pyogenes* and enteropathogenic *E. coli* are bacteria which may cause problems in neonatal units.

Nurses in neonatal units must be aware of how to handle and intercept faecal-oral transmission of pathogens. An outbreak of diarrhoea can rapidly lead to dehydration of the neonates, sometimes with fatal results. Prior to 1972, hexachlorophene was regularly used to bath infants. Brain damage in rats has been shown to be associated with a high serum hexachlorophene level in these animals. Since the restriction of 3% hexachlorophene in the bath water of neonates has been imposed, there has been an increase in the incidence of staphylococcal lesion in the neonatal units. These outbreaks are mainly related to skin infections.

Theoretically, no nurse with diarrhoea, no nurse who carries staphylococci, should attend to neonates. Gowning, gloving, masking and meticulous hand washing are routine in good neonatal units.

GENERAL REMARKS

Organisms responsible for nosocomial infection can be endogenous, derived from the patient's own flora, or exogenous derived from other patients, the staff or the environment.

Spread by direct contact can be decreased by:

(a) Adequate hand washing — Hands should be washed under a stream of running water using a good quality soap or an appropriate antiseptic. Care must be taken not to recontaminate one's hands on closing the tap. Elbow taps are specially provided to eliminate this problem.

(b) Gloves — these separate the skin of the hand with its residual bacteria from direct contact with the patient and his lesion.

(c) Gown — Disposable gowns are better than the sterilized linen ones. Contamination of the patient's side of the gown due to penetration of organisms from the wearer's clothing and skin, increases with the length of time the gown is worn.

Spread by indirect contact can be limited by:

(a) The use of disposable equipment which is packed in a sterile packet prior to use. Disposable equipment must only be used once and then disposed.

(b) Microbiological checks should regularly be made on vacolitres, autoclaved equipment and any other so-called 'sterile' instruments.

(c) Regular checks on the efficiency of the disinfectant should be made — 'in-use' testing is important.

(d) Bedpans, sputum mugs and other contaminated equipment should be washed-pasteurized.

(e) Baths, basins and toilets should be mechanically cleaned prior to the use of a disinfectant.

Droplet spread can be curtailed by:

(a) The efficient use of masks. Masks are worn covering both the nose and the mouth.

(b) Patients with infections spread by droplets may be isolated in cubicles with high walls.

(c) Laminar air flow is an expensive technique used to decrease the spread of organisms by droplets in leukaemia chemotherapy units.

(d) Patients with respiratory diseases, e.g. plague, pneumonia, tuberculosis, must be diagnosed early and not be put on a respirator in a general ward as this can lead to widespread dissemination of the organism.

Hospitals harbour many organisms. Counts of 10^8 organisms per millilitre are commonly found in excretions under standard hospital conditions. The role of the nursing staff in the control and prevention of nosocomial infections cannot be over emphasised. Hands are perhaps the major tool in hospital cross-infection!

Regular use of an antibiotic results in the selection of organisms resistant to that drug. The antibiotic exerts selective pressure on the bacterial population. Bacteria sensitive to the antibiotic are killed while those resistant to the drug survive and flourish. Resistant organisms are selected. On removal of the antibiotic these organisms are no longer at an advantage. If their resistance is due to a plasmid, i.e. an extra-chromosomal piece of genetic material which codes for resistance, they may now be at a metabolic disadvantage when competing with a bacterium lacking this plasmid.

Broad spectrum antibiotics should only be used in selected specified situations. Their routine use should be restricted.

THE CONTROL OF INFECTIONS SPREAD BY THE FAECAL-ORAL ROUTE

The source of the organism may be food. Kitchen staff may be carriers of typhoid or hepatitis A. The food may have been contaminated prior to reaching the hospital kitchen. Foodhandlers, food processing machines and packagings are all subject to public health control. The food may have started as a contaminated product, e.g. the duck or hen laying an egg may contaminate the egg with salmonella.

Adequate refrigeration with the maintenance of a cold chain will prevent the multiplication of any organisms which may be present. Cooking will kill most organisms; it will not inactivate certain enterotoxins. Cooked food should be eaten while still hot.

The type of organisms important in the spread of gastro-intestinal diseases is the same in hospital as in other institutions and at home. Pathogens include salmonella, shigella, enteropathogenic *E. coli*, rotavirus and hepatitis A virus. Their mode of spread is faecal-oral. Faecal contamination of food can be direct, or by fomites. The organisms are ingested with the food.

The role of the nurse in combating spread of faecal-oral infections includes adequate gloving and gowning when handling a patient admitted for gastro-intestinal infection. His excreta should be disposed of with the utmost care. Adequate disinfection and washing of hands on leaving the sickroom is imperative.

Nurses should not smoke on duty — not only do they run all the risks of the smoker in the general population, they also run the risk of introducing patient's enteric pathogens into their mouths. No nurse suffering from diarrhoea should handle the patient's food.

Equipment used in the nursing of one patient must not be used to spread organisms to other patients. Thermometers used on patients with infectious hepatitis should not be used on non-infected patients. Eating utensils and excreta receptacles should be sterilized and not merely disinfected. Disposable equipment should be used, disinfected and discarded.

SUMMARY
   (1) Nosocomial infections depend on the dissemination of organisms in hospitals. Nurses must be aware of the importance of person-to-person spread of organisms and must be trained to minimize this problem.
   (2) Surveillance by a hospital infection committee of the organisms present in the units, their modes of spread and their antibiotic resistance, gives the hospital administration a picture of infection control in their hospital. Microbiological surveillance of fomites, e.g. catheters and fluids, should be regularly performed.

NURSING — A HAZARDOUS OCCUPATION?

Nursing staff are in contact with sick patients. Many of these patients were admitted because of an infection, others were admitted for another reason. Nurses tend to be a healthy breed with intact host defences — the danger of them acquiring an infection is therefore lower than that of many of their sick patients. Nurses do, however, have close contact with patients and their excreta, e.g. bedpans, sputum mugs. Due to their increased exposure they are more at risk of acquiring an infection than a member of the general public.

The time of maximum danger for the nursing staff is the period between admission of the patient and the diagnosis of the disease. During this period special precautions are seldom taken. Danger of infection decreases as staff take adequate precautions and the condition, if amenable to specific therapy, is treated.

Organisms which may prove a danger to nursing staff are hepatitis A and B viruses. Hepatitis A virus causes infectious hepatitis and is spread by the faecal-oral route. Hepatitis B is spread in blood and blood products. A member of the nursing staff may become infected by introduction of this virus directly into a skin lesion or into the eye by an aerosol spray. Hepatitis B is capable of causing serious infections using the conjunctiva as the portal of entry.

Nurses also run the risk of acquiring syphilis in an unusual fashion. Skin lesions of secondary syphilis or blood from the syphilitic patient may both contain viable treponema. These spirochaetes may infect the nurse by penetrating a minor skin lesion or mucous membrane. Nurses are warned against biting nails and sucking thumbs when on duty.

From sputa nurses may acquire tuberculosis. From faeces they may acquire shigella dysentery, cholera or typhoid.

Nursing staff in children's hospitals are particularly at risk of exposure to the viral diseases of childhood. Chicken-pox, mumps and measles are all more severe in adults than in children. Mumps in adults may cause sterility. All these viral diseases are associated with an increased incidence of central nervous system complications in adults.

In spite of this list of risks to which members of the nursing profession are exposed, few of their number become ill. Perhaps this is in part due to their knowledge of the control and prevention of spread of microbial diseases!

Table XXXVIII

DISEASES REQUIRING ISOLATION OF THE PATIENT

Diphtheria
Smallpox
Typhoid
Open pulmonary tuberculosis
Measles
Whooping cough } N.B. in children's wards

TREATMENT, PREVENTION AND CONTROL OF INFECTIOUS DISEASES

Prevention can be approached at three levels:

(*a*) At the level of Man by —
   (i) Immunization;
   (ii) Health education;
   (iii) Early diagnosis and treatment.

(*b*) By control and elimination of vectors of disease.

(*c*) In the reservoir host.

Control can be implemented by —
   (i) Applying the principles used in prevention;
   (ii) Active treatment of the disease;
   (iii) Contact tracing.

PREVENTION AND CONTROL OF INFECTIOUS DISEASES

Prevention consists of measures taken to prevent the development of disease in an area. A receptive area is an area in which conditions are suitable for introduction and maintenance of disease. An area where there are anophelene mosquitoes and human hosts is an area which is receptive for malaria. Introduction of plasmodia into this area can lead to the establishment of a malaria endemic or epidemic area. Rivers and streams with water temperatures of above 5°C throughout the year are potential snail habitats. One man's excreta containing schistosome ova in a stream with snails of a susceptible genus, can lead to the introduction of bilharzia in that area. The introduction of one individual incubating variola into a susceptible population can result in deaths from smallpox in that area.

Prevention constitutes those measures adopted in order to protect against the introduction of disease into any one of these areas. Measures include vaccination and the screening of individuals and vehicles entering a receptive from an endemic area. Prevention is of value not only in the global public health scene, it is also of value to the individual.

Hospitals could be converted into death traps if measures were not employed to prevent infection of sick patients, e.g. by the infusion of contaminated fluids, the introduction of soiled catheters. The use of sterile equipment in hospitals is essential. Cross infection, e.g. from the typhoid or cholera patient, could wreak havoc in the absence of strict aseptic technique. Hospitals depend heavily on sterilization and disinfection procedures to prevent the spread of organisms and disease. The use of prophylactic antibiotics in selected cases is also a tool in the prevention of disease, e.g. the patient who has already had one attack of rheumatic fever with cardiac involvement cannot afford to risk further damage to his heart valves. This patient is a candidate for prophylactic antibiotics in order to prevent further disease.

Control is the overall term for measures employed in keeping disease at as low a level as possible. Control may employ similar measures to those used in prevention, but in slightly different situations. An area endemic for polio may control the disease by vaccination using an attenuated strain of the virus. This is an attempt to prevent infection with the wild strain of the virus which can result in paralytic poliomyelitis. The same is true of rubella, rubeola and mumps vaccination. Malaria can be controlled by the early treatment of patients, by spraying of insecticides to kill adult mosquitoes and by spreading oil on water in which mosquito larvae are developing. Successful attempts to interrupt the malaria transmission cycle results in control of the situation. Epidemics may be prevented. In areas where pathogenic organisms are concentrated, such as hospitals, spread is prevented and the situation controlled by aseptic measures. Early specific treatment, e.g. the use of antibiotics, adequate sanitation and measures controlling food and water hygiene, all constitute methods employed in the control of disease.

Prevention of disease in the individual may be achieved by:

(a) Not exposing that individual to the organism. This is not always possible.

(b) If the individual is likely to be exposed to the organism, the following measures may be implemented:

    (i) Host conditions can be made unfavourable for colonization by the pathogen. Good nutrition and avoidance of interference with the mechanical, chemical and especially the microbial barrier will assist attaining this objective.

   (ii) Active immunization — The type of vaccination or inoculation will determine the duration and extent of protection.

  (iii) Passive immunity — The neonate has a transfusion of immunoglobulins from the mother. Hyperimmune gamma globulin is available and will afford the individual temporary protection.

  (iv) Prophylactic chemotherapy — this should only be practised in specific situations.

Control — this is an attempt to expose the individual to no, or at worst, a minimal number of organisms. It requires a knowledge of the route and mode of spread of the organism as well as a knowledge of aseptic technique.

Examples include the use of masks to prevent droplet spread, the washing of hands and the hygienic handling of food and water to prevent ingestion of pathogens. The use of sterile gloves will prevent spread by direct contact and the use of insecticide sprays and mosquito nets will decrease exposure to arthropod vectors. The control of disease in a population also requires early treatment of and the tracing of all individuals who have had contact with the patient.

IMMUNIZATION

The aim of immunization is to achieve active protection of the individual against a realistic biological challenge infection. Protection is thus related to the dose and the virulence of the challenge organism. Not all vaccines are capable of fulfilling this criterion, e.g. typhoid inoculation only protects against exposure to a relatively low dose of *Salmonella typhi.*

Immunization is indicated (*a*) when a disease is caused by an organism with a high attack rate, or (*b*) when incapacitating clinical disease is produced. Infection by an organism may result in —

(i) loss of working hours, e.g. influenza is an economically crippling disease;

(ii) a significant morbidity — polio and meningitis may result in permanent sequelae;

(iii) death — the mortality rate of different diseases varies, e.g. pneumonic plague has almost a one hundred percent mortality.

Immunization may be available to the whole population, e.g. polio, smallpox; or it may be reserved for certain selected population groups. The selected population group is selected on the basis of 'high risk' as the determining criterion. Elderly people with respiratory and cardiac disease are selectively immunized against influenza which, in this group, is often a fatal disease. Females are selectively immunized against rubella — german measles can cause foetal abnormalities if contracted in early pregnancy. Vaccines available to the general population may in certain cases be legally required, e.g. smallpox and yellow fever are obligatory if one wishes to travel to certain areas. Other vaccines are optional, e.g. cholera immunization.

The time or optimal period for immunization varies according to the condition against which the vaccine is being used. Immunization against yellow fever is only required prior to travel involving entry into a yellow fever endemic area. Smallpox vaccination is given free of charge to residents living in endemic or high risk areas at the age of 12 months. Travellers entering or leaving an endemic smallpox area must produce evidence of having been vaccinated during the last 3 years. Protection against certain diseases is recommended just before the maximum morbidity period associated with acquisition of that disease, e.g. immunization against rubella in the female and against mumps in the male is recommended just before puberty. Girls do not become pregnant before puberty, boys do not develop mumps orchitis before puberty.

Certain vaccines are readily available to the public. These include immunization against polio, yellow fever, smallpox, rubella and mumps. Immunization against the following bacterial diseases is also available — whooping-cough, diphtheria, tetanus and tuberculosis. Vaccines against influenza, pneumococci and meningococci are available but only used if specifically indicated.

TYPES OF IMMUNIZATION

The principle underlying the use of an immunization programme is based on the knowledge that the host is capable of producing an immune response if exposed to an antigenic substance. In the case of vaccines, the antigen is derived from the pathogenic organism against which resistance is desired. Success in immunization depends on:

  (i) The correct choice of antigen — ideally the antigen to which the individual is exposed should be the factor endowing the organism with virulence, e.g. tetanospasmin in the case of *Cl. tetani*.

  (ii) The ability of the host to respond with an appropriate immune response.

A number of different vaccines are used. They can be divided into the following groups on the basis of their preparation:

(*a*) *The whole organism is used*

  (i) The killed organism is used when vaccines are produced against plague, cholera, whooping-cough and sometimes influenza.

  (ii) Live attenuated organisms are used against tuberculosis, polio, measles and german measles. Attenuation of an organism is achieved by growing that organism on an unfavourable medium.

Polio is a neurotrophic virus. Attenuation of this virus can be achieved by growing it on a succession of monkey kidney tissue cultures. This medium lacks nerve tissue and therefore poliovirus particles without selectivity for nervous tissue are favoured. The attenuated poliovirus which is then used to immunize human populations has lost its selectivity for nervous tissue.

(*b*) *Extracts of the organism may be used*

  (i) Secretory products, e.g. exotoxins may be extracted and treated. Toxoids are antigenically unchanged, biologically inactivated, toxins. A toxin may lose its potency on treatment with formalin. Formalin treated toxin retaining its antigenic site may be used in an immunization programme as a toxoid.

  (ii) Capsular or cell wall extracts. The virulence of the pneumococcus is directly related to its ability to resist phagocytosis. Neutralization of the anti-phygocytic ability of this organism renders it harmless. Immunization against pneumococci involves the use of an extract of the organism's capsule.

When there are different antigenic types of a virulence factor produced, the protection afforded by immunization is limited to the antigenic type used in the vaccine. Meningococci are classified into types A, B, C, D, W, X, Y and Z. Immunization with an extract from *N. meningitidis* type A will protect the individual against meningitis caused by type A, but it will not protect the individual against infection by any of the other types. A similar situation exists in the use of pneumococcal vaccine — there are over 82 different capsular types of pneumococci.

Certain problems have been encountered in the use of vaccines:

A. *The live vaccines*
This affords the individual better immunity than a killed vaccine. There

is, however, the risk that the organism may regain its virulence. In the case of BCG (the live attenuated mycobacterium vaccine), immunity is conferred on the individual as long as the organisms remain viable. Should the individual require steroids or other immunosuppressive therapy during this period, his defences may be sufficiently impaired to permit the inoculated mycobacterium to cause clinical disease.

Storage of live vaccine, e.g. measles, mumps or rubella should be at 4°C and less. These viruses are quickly killed at high temperatures or by exposure to sunlight. Oral polio virus vaccine should be stored at -10°C.

Certain live virus vaccines may have their colonization interfered with by other viruses. The oral live polio vaccine may fail to colonize the intestinal tract of a child when other enteroviruses are present in the intestine. Successful administration of the polio vaccine therefore requires more than one exposure to the vaccine.

B. *The killed or extracted vaccines*

No danger of infection by this material exists, no risk of infection in a host with impaired defences need be feared. The individual does, however, require a larger initial inoculum followed by multiple subsequent inoculations in order to establish good immunity. Immunity wanes after a number of years and boosters are necessary.

THE HOST RESPONSE TO IMMUNIZATION

The host response varies according to —

(*a*) the route of administration;

(*b*) the antigen.

If immunization is desired, a more appropriate host defence is illicited if the route of administration of the antigen is similar to that in natural infection. Immunization against, e.g. a respiratory tract pathogen is best achieved by inhalation, against gastro-intestinal tract infection by ingestion, of the antigen. Local immunity is then stimulated and IgA antibodies are excreted in the appropriate local secretions. If the vaccine is administered parenterally, local immunity is not enhanced and the host's antibody protection against the antigen is predominantly in the IgG fraction. Protection against influenza is better achieved by local exposure of the respiratory tract to the vaccine than by parenteral administration. Parenteral cholera or polio immunization leads to IgG anitbody production. This may protect the individual from disease but it does not prevent colonization by the virulent organism. Individuals who have been immunized against cholera may still be carriers of the organism. In theory an oral vaccine may prevent the carriage of wild strains of an organism.

The structure of certain organisms is subject to frequent variation. Immunization against such organisms will not be long-lasting. The organism which is known to excel at antigenic variation is the influenza virus. The frequency with which the organism achieves antigenic change affects the duration of immunity.

Table XXXIX
IMPORTANT VACCINES

VACCINES	TYPE OF VACCINE*	ORGANISM	DISEASE	COMMENT
Vaccines against bacterial organisms				
TAB	killed	*Salmonella typhi, S. paratyphi* A and B	typhoid enteric fever	T — moderately effective A, B — of no value
Cholera	killed	*Vibrio cholerae*	cholera	Protective in ±50% of individuals Immunity lasts for 3-6 months
DWT	toxoid	*Corynebacterium diphtheriae*	diphtheria	Boosters required
	killed	*Bordetella pertussis*	whooping-cough	
	toxoid	*Clostridium tetani*	tetanus	
BCG	live	*Mycobacterium tuberculosis*	tuberculosis	Single exposure protective for 8 years
Plague	killed	*Yersinia pestis*	plague	Only effective against bubonic plague
Brucella	live, attenuated	*Brucella abortus*	brucellosis	Used for cattle
Pneumococci	capsular polysaccharide antigen	*Strept. pneumoniae*	meningitis, pneumonia	Numerous different capsular types
Meningococci	capsular polysaccharide antigen	*N. meningitidis* types A and C	meningitis	Experimental stage
Vaccines against rickettsiae				
Typhus	live formalized antigen	*R. prowazeki*	epidemic typhus	Boosters every 6 months Live experimental
	formalized antigen	*R. rickettsiae*	Rocky Mountain spotted fever	

Table XL — *Continued*

Vaccines against viruses

VACCINE	TYPE OF VACCINE	ROUTE ADMINISTERED†	DISEASE	COMMENT
Rubella‡	live	s/c	german measles	Indicated in prepubertal females
Mumps	live	s/c	mumps	Indicated in prepubertal males
Rubeola	live	s/c	measles	Indicated in malnourished populations
Vaccinia	live	i/d	smallpox	Required by WHO for specific travel
Yellow fever	live	s/c or i/d	yellow fever	Reimmunization required after 8-10 years
Polio	live	oral	poliomyelitis	Trivalent vaccine — poliovirus types 1, 2, 3
Influenza	killed	s/c	influenza	Economic losses decreased
	live	inhaled		
Rabies	killed	s/c	rabies	Prepared in rabbit brain — neuroparalytic accident Duck egg vaccine also available

Key:

*vaccine preparation — live — live attenuated
killed — killed whole organism
toxoid — formalin treated toxin; biologically inactive

†s/c — sub-cutaneous   i/d — intra-dermal

‡may be given as a combined vaccine

The antigen to which the host is exposed may illicit either a predominantly humoral or cellular response. It is well recognised that a humoral response can be illicited and maintained by repeated exposure to killed organisms or products of these organisms.

A relatively long period elapses between first exposure to an antigen and antibody production to that antigen. The time lapse after primary exposure to bacterial antigens is of the order of 10 to 14 days. The first antibodies produced after parenteral injection are IgM, later these are replaced by a predominantly IgG antibody response. On second and subsequent exposure to the antigen, the time lapse between exposure to the antigen and antibody production is decreased, antibodies with a higher affinity for the antigen are produced, higher concentrations of antibody are produced and the duration of antibody production is prolonged. Immunization programmes against, e.g. diphtheria or tetanus, involve three successive exposures to the antigen at six weekly intervals. This is followed by a booster dose 12 to 18 months later. Repeated exposures are essential for —

(i) Better quality antibody production;
(ii) Larger quantities of antibody;
(iii) A longer duration of protection;
(iv) A swifter response by the host on re-exposure to the antigen in the form of the pathogenic organism.

Passive immunity may be achieved by infusion of antibodies into a susceptible individual; this gives the individual immediate but short-lived immunity.

The success of an immunization programme may be assessed in the laboratory by measuring the serum antibody levels attained on completion of the immunization course. Success of an immunization programme may also be assessed by the absence of the disease against which the population has been immunized.

Protection by cell mediated immunity appears to require the presence of a viable organism. Protection against tuberculosis using the BCG vaccine is achieved by stimulation of the cell mediated immune system. The time lapse between exposure and the development of immunity is longer than that of the humoral system. The efficiency of the immunization, the take, can be assessed by performing a tuberculin skin test (e.g. a Heaf or Mantoux test). The tuberculin test becomes positive 4-6 weeks after successful BCG immunization. No repeated exposure to the BCG vaccine is required in the next few weeks or months — in fact it is contra-indicated. Immunity to tuberculosis persists for as long as the mycobacterium inoculated remains viable. Immunity induced by successful BCG immunization lasts for 5 to 8 years.

Certain vaccines may be administered during pregnancy, e.g. yellow fever, tetanus. Rubella, mumps and smallpox should only be given after the infant is born.

Immunization is a powerful tool in the prevention of disease in communities and individuals. In those instances where immunization protects against clinical disease but does not prevent subclinical infection, carrier states may result. In such cases immunization is of value to the individual, but it fails to prevent introduction of disease into the community.

Table XL
AN IMMUNIZATION SCHEDULE

PRIMARY INNOCULATION	AGE RECOMMENDED FOR ADMINISTRATION
BCG	Given any time after birth.
DWT (against diphtheria, whooping-cough and tetanus)	Administered from the age of 3-6 months; 3 doses given at 6 weekly intervals
Oral polio	From 3 months (3 doses of triple vaccine)
Rubeola	From 9 months
Vaccinia	From 1 year
BOOSTERS	
DWT	18 months
DT, polio, vaccinia	5 years

INTERNATIONAL TRAVEL
Vaccination against smallpox and immunization against yellow fever and cholera may be required.

STERILIZATION AND DISINFECTION

Sterilization is the process whereby all micro-organisms and their spores are removed or destroyed. Disinfection is an attempt to remove or destroy all pathogenic organisms. Disinfection does not usually result in the destruction of bacterial spores.

If the techniques for sterilization do not conform to the stringent criteria required, the result may be disinfection rather than sterilization. It is essential that certain articles be sterile, e.g. intra-venous and urinary catheters. Other equipment may only require disinfection, e.g. washbasins, baths. Patients who harbour particularly pathogenic organisms, e.g. hepatitis virus, shigella, should have all the articles with which they have had contact adequately sterilized before these are permitted to be re-introduced into general circulation.

Sterilization is an all or none process. If all living micro-organisms have been killed then the object is sterile. If just one organism has survived the sterilization process then that object has been disinfected and not sterilized. 'Partially sterile', or 'almost sterile' are meaningless phrases.

METHODS FOR ELIMINATING OR DECREASING A MICROBIAL POPULATION

I. Adequate washing

Whatever the article, the first step in preparation for sterilization or disinfection is adequate mechanical cleansing. Sputum mugs, bedpans and all objects with organic wastes should first be mechanically cleaned. Adequate washing achieves a giant step in the right direction — up to 90%

of micro-organisms can be removed by this method. Elbow grease, soap and water have, on occasion, in selected circumstances, been shown to achieve results equivalent to cleaning with various disinfectants. Adequate mechanical cleaning can achieve better results than abuse of chemical disinfectants. The first rule in hospital hygiene should therefore be adequate mechanical cleaning. An exception to this is found when dealing with highly lethal organisms. Here it is advisable to kill the organism first!

II. Heat/pasteurization

Two forms of heat are available — moist heat and dry heat. Moist heat is capable of better penetration and hence is more effective than dry heat. Moist heat may kill the microbes by denaturing their enzymes and coagulating their proteins. Moist heat can effectively sterilize at a temperature of 121°C after exposure for 10 to 30 minutes.

Dry heat, because it penetrates less well than moist heat, requires a higher temperature and a longer period of exposure. Dry heat at a temperature of 160°C for 60 minutes will achieve sterilization. Organic material, e.g. paper or cotton-wool, char at this temperature. Dry heat is used in hot air ovens.

The effect of heat is therefore dependant on —
  (i) humidity;
  (ii) duration of exposure;
  (iii) the temperature achieved and maintained.

Death rate of organisms = temperature x time.

Prolonged exposure at lower temperatures may achieve similar results to shorter exposure at higher temperatures. This statement is true over a certain temperature range.

The autoclave — sterilization by heat

Articles requiring sterilization are often autoclaved. The autoclave is an elaborate pressure-cooker. In the autoclave, pressure is used to increase the temperature above that achieved by boiling water at normal atmospheric pressure. The influence pressure has on raising the temperature of boiling water can be easily demonstrated by boiling water at sea level and 1 800 metres (6 000 feet) above sea level. Water boils at a temperature of 100°C at sea level; it boils at approximately 94,5°C at 1 800 metres. In the autoclave, an increase in pressure of 1,2 kilograms per square centimetre (151 lbs/sq. inch) above atmospheric pressure at sea level will lead to an increase in the temperature of boiling water to 121°C. An increase in pressure of one atmosphere at sea level will therefore increase the temperature to 121°C.

The air in the autoclave can be removed either by 'downward displacement', i.e. the air is displaced by an inflow of steam, or, it may be pumped out in a 'high vacuum' autoclave. The latter type of autoclave does not have the problems of air pockets and a drier load is less likely to become contaminated. All sterile articles which are damp after autoclaving must be thoroughly dried in sterile cabinets.

The requirements for surgical sterilization are:

121°C x 18 minutes

or

115°C x 45 minutes

It must be noted that the exposure time quoted does not include heating up time.

The load to be sterilized must be kept at the temperature stated for the time period given. Viral susceptibility to heat varies, e.g. mumps and measles viruses are inactivated at room temperature. Many other viruses are destroyed at 60°C x 30 minutes. There are exceptions to this rule — hepatitis B virus is viable after being exposed to 60°C for 10 hours. Most vegetative bacteria are killed after 10 minutes at 50-65°C. Spore forms of fungi are less resistant than those of bacteria. Many, but not all clostridial spores are killed at 100°C after 10 minutes. The standard for surgical sterilization must thus be at a higher temperature, or for a longer duration, than those quoted to ensure killing of even the most resistant organisms.

It is necessary to have a means of controlling and checking the efficiency of sterilization. Two methods are popularly employed:

(*a*) Steri-tape is adhesive tape impregnated with strips of heat sensitive chemicals.

If these chemicals are exposed to an adequate temperature for a sufficiently long time, the strips change to a uniform black colour. If the steri-tape fails to change colour, or change occurs in a patchy distribution, one can conclude that the load is probably not sterile or that the steri-tape is defective. If the steri-tape is a uniform black colour after autoclaving, the conclusion is not that the load is sterile, but that the temperature and duration of exposure were sufficient to have caused a chemical reaction in the steri-tape. With fresh, accurate steri-tape such a change is only achieved under conditions which will destroy all living micro-organisms. Steri-tape is thus used as a reference standard. It is easy to use and gives an immediate indication of dysfunction during the sterilization procedure. Steri-tape is part of everyday life in a hospital.

(*b*) The biological control is an additional safeguard. This should be used at regular intervals in order to keep a microbiological check on the efficiency of sterilization.

Spores of a Gram-positive aerobic bacillus — *Bacillus stearothermophilus* — are introduced into the autoclave amongst the equipment to be sterilized. These spores remain viable after exposure to high temperatures. They are selected as a biological control because they are non-pathogenic heat resistant spores. These spores are destroyed at 121°C if exposed for

12 minutes. After autoclaving the spores are incubated under optimal laboratory conditions. If they fail to germinate after 48 hours it may be concluded that the load with which these spores were autoclaved is sterile.

Each load autoclaved should be checked by the steri-tape method; each week at least one load should, in addition, be checked by the biological control method.

Disinfection with heat

Heat disinfection plays an important role in laundering soiled linen. In most cases 65°C for 10 minutes will suffice. In the case of hepatitis virus when the linen and other equipment cannot be sterilized or discarded, then disinfection at 93°C for 10 minutes has been suggested.

Certain precautions are necessary when using heat:
  (i) The article being disinfected or sterilized must not be damaged by high temperatures. This is especially true when moist heat is being used.
  (ii) Only 'clean' articles should be pasteurized. Organic matter should be scrubbed or soaked away from any piece of equipment which is to be sterilized.
  (iii) When tubing is being sterilized, care must be taken not to trap air inside the tubing. This leads to inadequate heating of certain areas of the tube.

Uses for heat are numerous — surgical and anaesthetic equipment perhaps head the list. HEAT IS CHEAP AND EFFECTIVE.

III. Ethylene oxide

Micro-organisms may also succumb on exposure to certain toxic gases — one of these gases is ethylene oxide. It is of value in the sterilization of large instruments which would be damaged if exposed to heat. Suction pumps and humidifiers, after being checked for mechanical soundness, are exposed to ethylene oxide gas. Respirometers and respirators are first sterilized and then checked for mechanical defects.

Ethylene oxide is a toxic substance. Equipment sterilized by ethylene oxide must spend a period in an aeration area prior to use. Plastic and rubber articles require 7 days, metal requires a 48 hour period in the aeration area. The use of ethylene oxide imposes an obligatory delay between use, sterilization and re-use. The hospital using ethylene oxide sterilization thus requires a large initial outlay to allow for this slow turnover of equipment.

IV. Chemical disinfection

Many experts feel that chemical disinfection should only be used when heat or gas cannot be used.

A number of factors must be considered when chemical disinfection is being employed:

1. The spectrum of disinfectant activity. Chemical disinfectants, like antibiotics, have a specific range of activity. Phenolics and hypochlorites have a broad spectrum and kill a wide range of different micro-organisms. Quarternary ammonium compounds (QAC) and chloroxylenol, the exception in the phenolic group, are narrow spectrum with their activity largely confined to destruction of Gram-positive cocci. Chloroxylenol not only fails to inhibit the growth of Gram-negative bacilli, it provides an ideal culture medium for pseudomonas. Gluteraldehyde and hypochlorites are good disinfectants against spores; the iodophors, routinely used in theatre when spore forming organisms are likely to be encountered, are a little less effective against spores. Acid-fast bacilli such as *M. tuberculosis* are sensitive to alcohols, formaldehyde and iodophors.

2. Chemical disinfectants are only optimally active under specified conditions:

(*a*) Inactivation of the disinfectants must be avoided. Organic matter, e.g. pus, sputum, faeces, can seriously impair the action of a number of disinfectants, e.g. chloroxylenol, iodophors and hypochlorites. The clear phenolics are only slightly inactivated. If disinfection of urine or sputum is required prior to cleaning the urinal or sputum mug, then these excreta should be mixed with one of the clear soluble phenolics. Rubber, cotton, cork and plastics seriously impair the action of QAC's and chlorhexidine.

Most disinfectant solutions require dilution to the correct concentration before use. Hard water may seriously inactivate chloroxylenol, chlorhexidine and the QAC's.

(*b*) A disinfectant must be used at the correct concentration. A too dilute disinfectant loses some of its activity; a too concentrated solution is expensive and may be less efficient. Absolute alcohol is a less bactericidal disinfective than 70% ethyl alcohol.

Fresh dilutions of disinfectant should be made every morning. Once diluted, a disinfectant may lose some of its activity if left to stand for long periods. 'Topping' up of disinfectants is an activity shunned by all good nurses. It is well to remember that the correct dilution of a disinfectant is accurately measured and not estimated by the colour or smell!

Points to remember are:

(i) Accurate dilutions are essential.

(ii) Topping up of solutions can lead to propagation of an error made days previously and result in an inactive disinfectant.

(iii) Dilutions should be made on the same day on which they are to be used — dilution with hard water in a plastic container can lead to loss of activity; minimise this loss by not preparing the disinfectant the night before.

(iv) Containers used for measuring the correct dilutions of a disinfectant should not be assumed clean. They should be regularly washed and always be free of organic matter.

Inactivated disinfectants can support the growth of micro-organisms.

(c) The exposure time: this varies for different disinfectants. Chlorhexidine and 70% alcohol are quicker acting than the iodophors. The time required for the disinfectant to destroy micro-organisms is also modified by:

  (i) The temperature — disinfectants are usually more active at a higher temperature.

  (ii) The dilution of the disinfectant — disinfectants act best at the correct dilution.

  (iii) The presence of organic or other inactivating material.

  (iv) The microbiological load.

(d) The mode of action of different disinfectants differs. Basically disinfectants are either bactericidal — capable of killing micro-organisms, or bacteristatic — capable of interfering with further multiplication of the organism. Bacteristatic disinfectants should only be used when no bacteria are present; they do not decrease the number of bacteria, they merely prevent this number from increasing.

Bactericidal disinfectants kill bacteria. The rate of killing is influenced by the initial bacterial population. The larger the initial microbial population, the longer will a bactericidal disinfectant take to achieve a satisfactory result.

The biochemical mechanism whereby a disinfectant affects microbe growth and multiplication depends on the chemical structure of the disinfectant, e.g. phenolics act by denaturing protein.

In the selection of chemical disinfectants one must bear in mind:

(a) The spectrum of action of the disinfectant.

(b) The clinical situation in which the disinfectant will be used, e.g. theatre walls or in a sputum mug. Is the disinfectant going to be exposed to inactivating substances?

(c) The correct dilution of the freshly prepared solution.

(d) The correct exposure time.

Chemical disinfectants are used in three broad situations:

(a) As antiseptics — on skin and mucous membrane.

(b) As local surface disinfectants.

(c) As general disinfectants — this includes the decontamination of objects prior to disposal or re-use.

ANTISEPTICS

These must be non-irritant and act against gram positive organisms. The skin has a natural flora which is resistant to change; it also has a transient flora which may be significantly altered by antiseptics. Hands and sites which are to be subject to surgery or manipulation are the major anatomical areas requiring disinfection.

Regular hand washing with hexachlorophene leads to a residual concentration of the antiseptic in skin glands. This residual action is only achieved by regularly exposing the skin to this antiseptic. Hexachlorophene has a narrow spectrum — its activity is against Gram-positive cocci. Theatre and possibly neonatal unit personnel are therefore good candidates for using hexachlorophene. The control of staphylococci and streptococci on the hands of these nurses may benefit their patients.

Immediately before an operation, the theatre staff assisting the surgeon should wash their hands in 3% hexachlorophene; the final rinse should be with an iodophor or chlorhexidine alcohol (hibicol) mixture.

For rapid disinfection of various skin and mucous membrane sites, e.g. the intended site of the surgical incision, the venepuncture site, bladder irrigation, an antiseptic which acts rapidly and has a broad spectrum is required. Chlorhexidine combined with 70% alcohol is an expensive broad spectrum antiseptic. It does not kill spores. Patients with peripheral vascular disease undergoing above knee amputations, or those undergoing bowel surgery, should be prepared using an iodophor. Iodophors kill spores. Clostridial spores are found in the bowel of the great majority of people.

SURFACE DISINFECTANTS

A relatively quick acting disinfectant is usually selected as exposure time may be limited, e.g. the operating table should be wiped with a disinfectant between cases. A broad spectrum of activity is desirable. All surfaces should be cleaned and be free of obvious organic matter before being treated with a surface disinfectant.

Floors, walls, baths, stainless steel, glass and plastic surfaces may all be cleaned using surface disinfectants. Surface disinfectants include hypochlorites, 70% alcohol and a chlorhexidine mixture with a detergent.

GENERAL DISINFECTANTS

This group of disinfectants should be broad spectrum, relatively resistant to inactivation by organic matter and need not necessarily be quick acting. Phenolics, excluding chloroxylenol, are good general disinfectants. Brand names include printol, sudol, stericol, etc.

In-use testing

Factories testing the efficiency of disinfectants do so under ideal conditions. In-use testing of disinfectants is of more immediate practical value. The in-use testing of a disinfectant tests the disinfectant in a specific clinical situation. It tests the disinfectant under conditions in which the disinfectant is being used. In-use testing tests the efficiency of the disinfectant, and it also tests the accuracy with which the solution is prepared. In-use testing reveals the usefulness of a disinfectant as it is made and used in the hospital ward or unit.

Without sterilization and disinfection, little success would be enjoyed in the prevention and control of infections in the hospital environment.

Mortality and morbidity would rocket with each surgical and invasive procedure. Thanks to advances in the field of disinfectants and sterilization, theatre technique has moved from the use of antiseptic to aseptic technique. Antiseptic technique permits the presence of a very limited number of 'non-pathogenic' organisms, aseptic technique excludes all micro-organisms.

SUMMARY

Methods available:

MECHANICAL CLEANING

STERILIZATION by —
- (i) Heat
- (ii) Ethylene oxide

DISINFECTION by —
- (i) Heat
- (ii) Chemical disinfectants
    - (*a*) antiseptics, e.g. hexachlorophene
    - (*b*) surface disinfectants, e.g. hypochlorites
    - (*c*) general disinfectants, e.g. phenols

Sterilization means the removal or killing of ALL micro-organisms. Disinfection means the removal of most of the organisms present — resistant forms include —
- (i) spores — use iodophor, gluteraldehyde;
- (ii) hepatitis B virus — use 2% gluteraldehyde, 10% formalin;
- (iii) *M. tuberculosis* — use formaldehyde, iodophor.

Don'ts in disinfection
- (i) Do not dilute the solution in an inaccurate manner. Never top-up an old solution.
- (ii) Do not use yesterday's disinfectant today. Make up fresh solutions daily.
- (iii) Do not clean sharp instruments by washing and then expect them to become sterile by storage in a disinfectant solution. All instruments should be sterilized and stored in sterile dry containers until they are required. The nurse who attempts to 'help' the surgeon who drops his favourite scalpel by picking it up from the floor and quickly dipping it into a disinfectant solution would be more worthily employed assisting the pathologist in the mortuary.
- (iv) Do not store nail and toilet brushes in pseudomonas culture media, viz. in chloroxylenol. Keep this antiseptic for use in situations where it is of value.
- (v) Do not allow organic matter to decrease the efficiency of the disinfectant being used.
- (vi) Do not re-use disposable equipment. Dispose of it!

THE USE OF ANTI-MICROBIAL AGENTS

Anti-microbial agents are chemical substances or drugs used to destroy or inhibit the growth of micro-organisms. There are two types of anti-microbial agents:

(*a*) those which are synthesised by micro-organisms — these are collectively called antibiotics;

(*b*) those which are synthesised in the laboratory by biochemists.

Anti-microbial agents may be further divided into two large groups on the basis of their ability to interrupt the life cycle of the organism:

(i) Bactericidal antibiotics (e.g. penicillin) kill or lyse the organism.

(ii) Bacteristatic anti-microbial agents (e.g. tetracycline) interfere with the metabolism and multiplication of the organism.

Anti-microbial agents are used to treat clinical disease. They may also, in specific circumstances, be used to prevent infection, or to prevent disease developing in individuals who have been exposed to an organism.

USE OF PROPHYLACTIC ANTI-MICROBIAL AGENTS

Anti-microbial agents should not be used for prophylaxis except in specific circumstances. The uncontrolled use of antibiotics can lead to:

(*a*) Superinfection, i.e. alteration of normal flora and overgrowth by fungi, e.g. candida and/or other pathogens.

(*b*) An increase in antibiotic resistant organisms.

Prophylactic antibiotics may be indicated in the following circumstances. Opinions differ in all the examples to be mentioned. Experts also differ in their choice of antibiotic and the dosage they recommend.

A. *A healthy host with a good immune response:*

(i) The contacts of patients admitted to hospital with meningococcal meningitis. Certain authorities believe that all contacts deserve prophylactic anti-meningococcal therapy. With increasing resistance against sulphonamides becoming evident amongst meningococci, the anti-microbial agents recommended are minocycline and rifampicin.

(ii) Women who have had contact with a male diagnosed as having gonorrhoea should be investigated for gonorrhoea. In the female this disease is often asymptomatic, isolation of the organism is often difficult. In the absence of adequate laboratory confirmation these women should be treated with a prophylactic penicillin injection.

(iii) Prior to bowel surgery the preparation of the intestine usually includes anti-microbial agents. Certain authorities feel that mechanical cleaning of the bowel is insufficient unless this is supplemented by anti-microbial therapy.

(iv) Chemo-prophylaxis against malaria is routinely used by people travelling in malaria endemic areas.

(v) Individuals who have had contact with plague victims are immediately and routinely given tetracyclines.

B. *Hosts with an altered immune response:*

  (i) *An unusual immune response* — Certain individuals who have had a *Streptococcus pyogenes* throat infection develop delayed sequelae some weeks later. Rheumatic fever can and often does leave residual heart damage. This damage is irreversible. Individuals who have once responded with cardiac damage to a streptococcal throat infection are likely to do so on subsequent occasions. Prophylactic penicillin in low doses will prevent reinfection with *Streptococcus pyogenes* and therefore it will prevent exacerbations or rheumatic fever.

  (ii) *An immature immune system* — The neonate lacks a fully competent immune system. He acquires maternal IgG by transplacental spread. Ophthalmia neonatorum is infection of the newborn baby's eyes by *N. gonorrhoeae* acquired by passage through the birth canal. Blindness can be prevented by early treatment of this condition. Females are often asymptomatic carriers of the organism. It is therefore routine practise for the baby to have silver nitrate or penicillin drops instilled into its eyes shortly after birth. Neonates who are premature and have survived for long periods in utero after the membranes have ruptured, who required instrument intervention and who passed through a genital canal which appears infected, are often put onto prophylactic anti-microbial therapy.

  (iii) *An impaired or depressed immune response* — Patients who demonstrate a positive tuberculin test should be placed on prophylactic INH (anti-tuberculous therapy) prior to institution of immunosuppressive therapy, e.g. steroids which may be indicated for a collagen disease. The patient who requires steroid therapy or who is a candidate for organ transplantation should therefore have a tuberculin test before such therapy is embarked upon.

  (iv) *Anatomical abnormalities which interfere with the superficial defence barrier* — A fractured base of skull leading to direct communication between the meningies and the ear, the sinuses and/or the exterior, is a potent danger. Pneumococci are normal commensals of the upper respiratory tract; if these organisms are transported to the meninges and central nervous system, meningitis may be followed by brain abscess. Certain workers advocate prophylactic antibiotics to intercept this postulated cycle.

Patients suffering from chronic bronchitis may be placed on chemoprophylaxis at certain times when the risk of an acute exerbacation is increased.

Patients with damaged heart valves, e.g. after rheumatic fever, due to atheromatous degeneration, a congenital defect, or after valve replacement, are all at risk of thrombi and organisms settling on these valves.

Individuals who have a known valvular defect who are subject to manipulations leading to bacteraemia, should only have these procedures performed under adequate antibiotic cover.

PRINCIPLES OF SPECIFIC ANTI-MICROBIAL THERAPY

The use of drugs in the treatment of infectious diseases is governed by certain basic principles. If all these principles are fulfilled a good and often rapid recovery can be predicted. If none of these criteria are met, the drug is of no value except as a placebo. It may even have deleterious side effects. Certain viral conditions are occasionally treated with placebos.

Specific therapy constitutes treatment using drugs which act directly and specifically against the infecting agent. Supportive therapy is not aimed at removing the organism; its purpose is to help the patient to feel better. The common cold is often treated with acetyl salicylic acid — this helps the patient to feel better but it may increase the number of viruses shed into the environment by that patient.

Basic guidelines for specific therapy

(*a*) The drug must be more toxic to the organism than to the host. The drug should act on the structures or metabolic pathways which differ between the host and the infecting organism, e.g.:

(i) Bacteria have an enzyme complement capable of converting para-aminobenzoic acid into folic acid. Mammalian cells lack this enzyme system. Anti-microbial agents, e.g. sulphonamides, can act on this enzyme system preventing the organism producing the folic acid it requires for normal metabolism and multiplication.

(ii) Ribosomes are found in both mammalian and bacterial cells. Their structure does, however, differ. Chloramphenicol and tetracyclines only interfere with protein synthesis on bacterial ribosomes.

(iii) Bacteria have cell walls composed of structural units foreign to man. Penicillin interferes with bacterial cell walls without in any way interfering with mammalian cell membranes. Fungi incorporate sterols into their cell membranes; man lacks these sterols. Anti-fungal agents which interact with the sterol component of the fungal cell wall may be used in the treatment of fungal disease.

Differential toxicity is of the utmost importance in the treatment of infectious disease. The aim of the therapy is the death of the organism without damage to the host. The greater the similarity of structure and function between the organism and host, the greater the toxicity to the host on treatment of the disease. Viruses and higher protist infections are more difficult to treat than infections caused by lower protists. Some drugs are bactericidal — they kill the organism; others are bacteristatic — these inhibit further multiplication of the organism. Bacteristatic anti-microbial agents depend on the host's defences for elimination of the organism.

(*b*) The following criteria must be fulfilled before anti-microbial therapy can be successful:

(i) The drug must reach the organism. Organisms hidden in the centre of necrotic lesions are protected against the drug. An abscess should therefore be drained and the remaining bacteria will be eliminated by the anti-microbial agent. Only an adequate blood supply will ensure delivery of the drug to an infected area. Intracellular organisms, e.g. *M. tuberculosis, M. leprae* and *Salmonella typhi* also enjoy a degree of protection against the penetration of drugs. Successful chemotherapy requires exposure of the organism to adequate blood levels of the appropriate anti-microbial agent.

The quantity of drugs administered, the frequency of administration and the route of administration all influence the blood level of the drug. It is the responsibility of the nursing staff to ensure that hospitalized patients get the anti-microbial agent prescribed by the doctor in the correct dose and at the correct intervals.

(ii) The drug must be active at the site occupied by the organism, e.g. changes in pH, or ion concentration may alter the efficiency of the drug.

(iii) The infecting organisms must be susceptible or sensitive to the drug being used. Certain organisms are naturally resistant to certain anti-microbial agents, e.g. *Bordetella pertussis* is resistant to penicillin. Certain organisms may be resistant due to their genetic complement — this resistance is chromosomal in origin. Induced resistance may occur amongst large groups of organisms, e.g. gram negative bacilli, by transfer of pieces of genetic material (plasmids). These plasmids are called R factors. R factors may be transferred from one group of bacteria to another.

Resistance to drugs may be due to:

(i) The organism being impermeable to the drug.

(ii) The organism may produce an enzyme capable of inactivating the anti-microbial agent.

(iii) The structure of the active site may be changed, e.g. the ribosome may be structurally altered so that the drug can no longer attach to its biochemical site of action.

(c) Drugs are more active against actively multiplying and metabolising organisms. This is not unexpected as anti-microbial agents frequently interfere with metabolic pathways, protein synthesis or cell wall structure. If the organisms are quiescent, they will not be utilizing many metabolic pathways, nor will they be producing many proteins and enzymes. Infections caused by *E. coli* with a generation time of approximately 20 minutes is cured in days and seldom weeks; infection caused by *M. tuberculosis* with a generation time of 20 hours is treated for weeks, months and sometimes years. The generation time of an organism is not the only factor determining the duration of therapy.

(d) The co-operation of the patient in the taking of the drug is always a great help.

It is essential that the correct anti-microbial agent be administered in an adequate dosage at correct intervals for a sufficient period of time.

The failure to respond to therapy

This may be due to one or more of the following reasons:

(a) The organism may be resistant to the drug, e.g. penicillin G is an excellent antibiotic in the treatment of infections caused by gram positive organisms, but has little effect on gram negative bacilli.

(b) The drug may be improperly administered, e.g. the route, dose or duration of administration may be incorrect.

(c) There may be a failure to use auxiliary therapy, e.g. an abscess is treated firstly by drainage and only secondarily with antibiotics.

(d) Host factors may complicate the picture, e.g. the host's defences may be impaired. The patient may have an anatomical defect, e.g. a urethral valve. The presence of a foreign body may interfere with drainage of an organ, e.g. stones in the gall bladder; or may interfere with the host's defences, e.g. asbestos in lung macrophages.

The abuse of anti-microbial agents

Antibiotics are too often resorted to when the clinician is in doubt. Anti-microbial agents should be used to treat infections and not to treat non-specific fevers. Viral infections are all too frequently treated with antibiotics.

Antibiotics must only be used for prophylaxis in specific circumstances. They must never be used in food preservation or animal feeds.

A broad spectrum anti-microbial agent must be avoided except in select cases. Tetracycline should only be used in diarrhoea if cholera has been diagnosed.

Complications due to anti-microbial chemotherapy

Chemotherapeutic agents are not without side effects. They must only be used in the treatment of organisms likely to succumb to them. The hepatic, renal, and haematological systems are often the systems first affected by excessive or inappropriate anti-microbial therapy. Certain of these drugs may lead to deafness, and/or dizziness due to effects on the ear or the VIII nerve. Peripheral neuritis is a common complication.

Oral broad spectrum anti-microbial agents are well known to alter the normal bowel flora, to interfere with the host's normal microbial barrier and permit superinfection in the gastro-intestinal tract.

HOSPITAL ANTIBIOTIC POLICY

Hospitals have a definite approach to the use of anti-microbial agents. This policy is aimed at giving the correct and cheapest anti-microbial agent to the patient; it is also aimed at reducing and controlling the emergence of hospital strains of antibiotic resistant organisms.

The policy

(a) Treat patients as outpatients whenever possible, e.g. avoid admission of patients with chronic urinary tract infection unless their clinical condition warrants hospitalization; the same is true of the chronic bronchitic.

(b) Discharge patients as soon as possible — aim at short hospital stays.

(c) Continual surveillance of antibiotic resistance in the hospital will lead to early detection of increased resistance to a certain anti-microbial agent. This drug should then be removed from use in the wards.

(d) Rotation of antibiotics, i.e. the use of antibiotics for limited periods, followed at a later date by the re-introduction of that antibiotic into hospital use, has been shown to lessen the resistance to that drug.

The use of anti-microbial agents:

(a) Full dose and short courses are recommended.

(b) Chronic infections are often treated with more than one drug simultaneously.

(c) Use a narrow spectrum antibiotic whenever feasible.

(d) Use only antibiotics when there are definite indications for their use.

Decrease introduction of infection by:

(i) The use of aseptic technique.

(ii) Local irrigation.

(iii) Local applications.

Table XLI

GUIDELINES TO ANTI-MICROBIAL THERAPY

ANTI-MICROBIAL AGENT	SUSCEPTIBLE ORGANISMS*	MAJOR SIDE EFFECT
PENICILLIN†	cocci, Gram-positive bacilli, spirochaetes	hypersensitivity
AMPICILLIN, AMOXY-CILLIN	shigella, haemophilus, *Strept. faecalis, Salmonella typhi*	see penicillin
TETRACYCLINE	mycoplasma, rickettsiae, chlamydia, *Vibrio cholerae*, *Neisseria gonorrhoea*, spirochaetes, brucella	Broad spectrum ... risk of superinfection, GIT upsets Not used in pregnant women
AMINOGLYCOSIDES e.g. streptomycin gentamycin kanamycin neomycin	Gram-negative bacilli	Renal and VIII nerve toxicity

Table XLI (*continued*)

ANTI-MICROBIAL AGENT	SUSCEPTIBLE ORGANISM	MAJOR SIDE EFFECT
CHLORAMPHENICOL	*Salmonalla typhi* *Haemophilus influenzae*	bone marrow depression
SULPHONAMIDES	Community acquired *E. coli* urinary tract infection Prophylaxis in case contacts of bubonic plague	allergy crystalluria
RIFAMPICIN, INH, ETHAMBUTOL, ETHIONA- MIDE, THIOCETAZONE, PYNAZINAMIDE, STREPTOMYCIN	*M. tuberculosis*	hepatic, neural
DAPSONE	*M. leprae*	
AMPHOTERICIN B GRISEOFULVIN	fungi	renal failure, GIT upsets, skin rashes GIT upsets
5-IODO-2'-DEOXYURIDINE	viruses	cytotoxicity

*In certain cases important exceptions may be found, e.g. *Strept. faecalis* is resistant to penicillin.

†In cases of penicillin hypersensitivity, use erythromycin in minor and cephalosporins in more serious infections.

Final choice of anti-microbial therapy depends on sensitivity testing and the patient's response.

Index